RETURNING FROM QINGCHENG MOUNTAIN

RETURNING FROM QINGCHENG MOUNTAIN

MELDING DAOIST PRACTICES INTO DAILY LIFE

WANG YUN

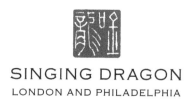

SINGING DRAGON

LONDON AND PHILADELPHIA

First published in Great Britain in 2022 by Singing Dragon,
an imprint of Jessica Kingsley Publishers
An Hachette Company

1

Copyright © Wang Yun 2022
Translated by the Modern Wisdom Translation Group

The right of Wang Yun to be identified as the Author of the Work has been asserted
by him in accordance with the Copyright, Designs and Patents Act 1988.

Front cover image source: Shutterstock®.

Disclaimer: The practice of *qigong* is intended to be a complementary therapeutic practice,
its primary goal being prevention of disease through the strengthening of the body's
immune and musculoskeletal systems, and the regulation of respiratory and circulatory
functions. It is not intended as a replacement for professional and timely medical care.
The reader is urged to consult a medical professional on any matter concerning their
health, and to follow the given diagnoses and prescriptions. Harking back to its classical,
poetical roots, the Chinese language relies heavily on figures of speech such as hyperbole
and metaphors, in order to evoke strong, multisensorial responses in the reader. While
rendered in English translation, some statements may seem definitive absolutes, they
are rather meant to convey the rhetorical strength of a given argument in the original;
they are to be taken for their suggestive, evocative power, rather than literally.

A CIP catalogue record for this title is available from the
British Library and the Library of Congress

ISBN 978 1 78775 896 4
eISBN 978 1 78775 897 1

Printed and bound by CPI Group (UK) Ltd, Croydon CR0 4YY

Jessica Kingsley Publishers' policy is to use papers that are natural, renewable, and recyclable
products and made from wood grown in sustainable forests. The logging and manufacturing
processes are expected to conform to the environmental regulations of the country of origin.

Jessica Kingsley Publishers
Carmelite House
50 Victoria Embankment
London EC4Y 0DZ

www.singingdragon.com

Contents

PART 2: PRACTICE GUIDE AND EXERCISES

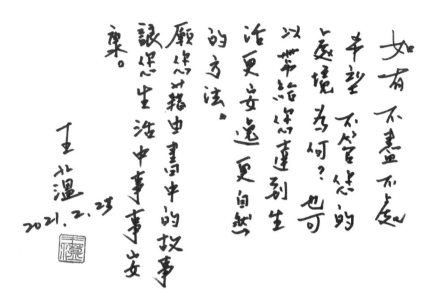

如有不盡不起
希望不管您的
之處境為何？也奇
以帶給您達到生
活更安逸更自然
的方法。
願您藉由書中的故事
讓您生活中事事安
康。

王北疆
2021.2.23

Though much may have been omitted, I hope that what I was able to recall can give you a way to be natural, healthy, and at peace with your life. Regardless of what circumstances you face, may you be like the figures from the stories within, and approach all things with a calm and steady head, and heart.

TRANSLATOR'S PREFACE

In the wake of the success of the first two volumes of the *Qingcheng Mountain* series, we have been overjoyed by the enthusiasm of our readers and humbled by the positive feedback.

Recent times have been challenging for the mind and body of many across the globe: while the situation has been unfortunately dire for many, it is with fortuitous timing that this series has been made available in English. Beyond the cultivation of health and vitality available to those who might practice the techniques within, there is also the broader prospect of glimpsing, daresay walking, the "Path of Immortals." The avenue brings the rare few—some whose stories you will find in this third installment—to surpass the limitations of the human body and mind, and reach states of rarefied physical and spiritual exaltation.

While Wang Yun is liberal in sharing these remarkable stories, both from history and from his own encounters, he always brings back the wonders of the Daoist path to the realm of the ordinary, to the playground of our spiritual experience: our daily life, and our mind.

The Practice Guide and Exercises in Part 2 of the present book presents the "12-Step Longevity Practice" and the "Eight Pieces of Brocade," both simple and straightforward exercise sets that can assist the practitioner in strengthening their body through promoting the circulation of *qi*[1] and blood, as well as maintaining the health of the tendons, ligaments, joints, and muscles. Yet the greater message of this book lies in the preponderance of the mind in governing our health and well-being. Indeed, it could be said that its essence—and that of Wang Yun's Daoist teachings in

---

1 氣: The vital force present in all living entities.

general—can be contained in one of its opening passages, namely "*qi* is the medicine of eternity, and the mind is the emissary of *qi*."

Among the trials the world has faced in recent times, the anxiety, depression, and plethora of mental issues that occur as a result of isolation and solitude stand at the forefront. It may seem paradoxical, then, to discover that solitude and retreat have been sought out by generations of spiritual seekers and practitioners as a source of inner discovery and even an essential tool for inner cultivation. It is thus our hope that the practices and worldview shared in this volume can bring appropriate assistance in such dire times, and help transform the angst and alienation that the current crisis has brought to the surface. We do firmly believe that these challenging times have granted us an opportunity to slow down and take the time to become acquainted with our breath and mind, as well as the space to discover the heritage of the Daoist tradition, experientially.

In the course of our own study and practice under Wang Yun, we have come to appreciate ever more the wisdom in his teachings, of cultivating the body's health through *qigong*,[2] but essentially of maintaining inner poise and relaxation as the foundation for sound health.

What we believed to be the concluding volume of the *Qingcheng Mountain* trilogy has, during the course of this translation, become but the third volume of an ongoing bestseller series on health cultivation. This news perhaps did not surprise as much as it delighted us: we have come to take in stride the gradual unveiling of a seemingly bottomless well of knowledge and experience, as well as Wan Yung's constant revelations that what we see as the end is perhaps just the beginning of a new chapter.

It is an honor and a privilege to study with such a teacher and

---

2 氣功: Literally "breath/air work" or "breath skill." In broad terms, the discipline, developed mostly in ancient China by Daoist practitioners, that focuses on the cultivation of the breath and internal *qi* to strengthen one's body and ensure long-lasting health. Its myriad exercises are the basis for all other internal/external martial arts of the Chinese tradition.

master, and we do hope that our present translation of his wonderful prose can lend you a glimpse into this fabulous Daoist master's heritage for the modern world.

PART 1

RETURNING FROM QINGCHENG MOUNTAIN

CHAPTER 1

Unifying Mind and *Qi*— the Secret of Success in Daoist Cultivation

My first year learning about the preliminary phases of Daoist meditation practices from *sifu*[1] was coming to a close. Around that time, *sifu* imparted something to me about how to proceed after entering a meditative state: the statement left a profound impression on me. Later, I verified the advice against a reference from the *Baopuzi*: this work addresses the cultivation of *qi* and the Daoist path of practice, and points to the ingestion of medicine as a means of obtaining longevity. But in fact, the "medicine" the text refers to is the principle of *qi* circulation, which can only be attained after receiving oral instruction.[2] If one knows the tricks of the technique, one can at least reach the stage of "gathering the small medicine."[3] However, attainment of the "big medicine"[4] depends on the seeker's basic aptitude or whether the seeker has an experienced master willing to teach them these techniques. Experienced practitioners are all quite clear that the most crucial element in obtaining great accomplishment in meditation and *qi* cultivation is to unify one's

---

1   師父: A respectful, commonly used epithet for one's teacher/master or for an elder with expertise in a certain field. We chose the *sifu* transliteration (rather than the standard pinyin *shifu*) to better match Wang Yun's own pronunciation.

2   竅訣 (*qiaojue*): A special tip given at the correct time in order to develop a student's practice. The term 口訣 (*koujue*) places emphasis on being spoken directly by a teacher. Both of these are translated in this book as "oral instruction."

3   採小藥 (*caixiaoyao*): The process whereby essence is transformed to *qi* in preparation for further practices.

4   大藥 (*dayao*): While the accumulation of small medicine (採小藥) is the collection and transmutation of essence to *qi*, collecting big medicine describes the transmutation of this *qi* into spirit.

mind and *qi*, the principle at the heart of this being "*qi* is the medicine of eternity, and the mind is the emissary of *qi*." If the mind and *qi* are in mutual support, then it is possible for the practitioner to obtain immortality. Before people become consumed with the worldly cares of tomorrow, before the corrupting influence of mundane, commercial life, the *qi* and blood within them flows naturally; however, ignorance and corruption gradually block the sources and channels, leading to stagnation of *qi* and blood. This is the genesis of a myriad illnesses. One needs oral instruction to once again open and connect the eight channels.

I still remember an oppressively hot summer evening from 1978, sometime around late June: twice a week, while visiting *sifu*'s residence in Yonghe, I would accompany him at a banquet. Although *sifu* maintained a low profile and lived hidden within the city, many admiring practitioners of the Dao would come from far away to seek him out. People came from abroad, from central and southern Taiwan; old comrades from his army days came; skeptic seekers came; people who knew him from his hometown long ago. Almost every night, two to three tables were laid out for the company; no one was ever turned away. *Sifu*'s manner on these occasions was like that of Meng Changjun (circa 3rd century BCE) from antiquity. I developed a deep admiration for his consistent demonstration of chivalry and hospitality. Among the visitors, there were no disciples of great prowess, none whom the master could rely on for their skill, as Meng Changjun relied on Feng Xuan. In any case, these visitors came from various places and walks of life. From celebrities to common laborers, they were all received by *sifu*, and he did not discriminate among them. He was thoroughly accommodating in his guidance of each seeker, and he rarely exhibited fatigue.

On a particular evening one weekend, two elders, whom *sifu* had known for many years, were present at dinner. One, a dual practitioner of Buddhism and Daoism, was Elder Lin, a man of profound insight. The other was an esteemed disciple of Elder Wang, the Daoist brother of *sifu*'s from years past when he lived in old Shanghai. Ten to twenty people were sitting around two old-style square tables with eight seats, sharing food and talk; I was humbled and fortunate to be among them. After everyone had eaten their fill, the elders began recounting events long past and martial arts tales from history; they even gave an abundance of valuable descriptions of critical events related to Daoist elders of lore. I benefited greatly from what they shared.

That night, among those present was one of Elder Wang's personal disciples, a Daoist priest by the surname Tong. He had come to meet and seek an audience with *sifu* for the first time. This priest was a fascinating character, and his every word shone with wit. Being around 70 years old, he had achieved some status as a practitioner and had seen and experienced a great deal.

It was said that he had followed Elder Wang for many years, and had heard from him many stories about the customs of old Shanghai, as well as apocryphal accounts of eccentric people's lives.

How was it that the topic of the evening turned to Beijing Opera? Perhaps because *sifu* would sometimes participate in casual performances, and on occasion, when he had spare time, people would present him with tickets to the theater. It may have been that Priest Tong had heard of *sifu*'s appreciation of theater, and thus to warm up the conversation had put forward this theme.

Priest Tong began: "I am Shanghainese, and therefore from an early age I began going to the theater with my mother and father to hear famous performers sing in the operas. My brothers, too, beginning in childhood, would spend a lot of time at the theater with my parents during the holidays—we knew the history of the opera industry's rise and fall as if it were written in the lines in our hands. My parents were also on familiar terms with some of the big names in the business, so once in a while we would join the amateur troupes in a performance. These experiences influenced my understanding of stage presence and vocal music. Because I was particularly interested in martial arts, I paid special attention to the skills related to warrior roles.

My childhood home was not far from Baiyun Temple, and

around the New Year holiday, my parents would often take the family elders and us children to Baiyun Temple to pray for blessings. At the temple there was a Daoist priest who acquired some solid training of *gongfu*.[5] Word had it that year in and year out, whether in winter or summer, he always wore the same simple robe, and otherwise owned nothing. He never wore any shoes, even on the coldest winter days when snowflakes swirled about him. Yet, curiously, he never seemed to tremble from the cold, nor would the color of his feet change. During summers, with the sun at its peak and beating down on him, he wore that same long robe. Sometimes I saw him perform Daoist rituals: wearing one of those traditional Daoist crowns on his head, he would perform the 'Steps of Yu,' tracing the star pattern of the Big Dipper with his hands and feet. The strangest thing was, not a single bead of sweat appeared as he performed the mystical dance; this astonished and puzzled many people.

It was also said that every year, this old priest would enter and remain in a meditative state for 100 days. During these periods he would observe the Daoist life-prolonging practice of abstaining from grains. He would, in fact, fast altogether. Day-to-day, he was careful with every type of reaction or expression; he didn't smile or speak. However, every year he would permit pilgrims and people he knew from the area to be inducted into the Daoist teachings. Because of his reputation, there was no end to the visitors; they waited in long queues to see him.

This old priest was on friendly terms with my father because they grew up in the same village. Perhaps owing to this, he took special notice of me. How was it that I was predestined to have such a bond with him? He would often pat me on the shoulder or affectionately pinch my cheeks; sometimes he even imparted a few nuggets of wisdom. In those years I was still quite young and had little experience in the ways of the world. I just thought of

---

5 功夫: Meaning "skill," applied to all kinds of fields of expertise. Often transliterated as *kungfu* or *kung-fu* in the West, it refers, somewhat incorrectly, to a particular style of Chinese external martial arts.

him as a compassionate old man who often put his hands on my shoulders—despite their strength, they were ever soft and warm, even in winter.

On holidays throughout the year, I would go with my older brother to stroll and look about inside the temple. On one such occasion, we serendipitously encountered the old priest just as he was emerging from his period of fasting and meditation. He gestured to my brother and me to approach. Pulling up a chair in the side chamber, the priest took a seat, and then spoke to me."

CHAPTER 2

"Sixteen Gold Ingots"—Each Word a Precious Treasure

Tong continued his story: "'I see within you the soul of a practitioner,' the old priest had said. 'In the future, you will encounter the teachings of the Dao. For now, I will impart a few strands of wisdom to you. If you rely on these words on your path of cultivation, then you will remain in good health. In days to come, you will entrust yourself elsewhere to another teacher, but what you receive here will not pose any conflict to this destiny.

In two years, you will face illness. The technique I will teach you now will come in handy, and you must apply it. You must brand it into your heart. Memorize and recite it. Practice a few times with me now: one inhalation facilitates rising; cycle the breath, return to the navel; one rise facilitates gulping; water and fire thus meet.'[1]

The old master taught me the technique, simultaneously explaining and demonstrating the breathing practice. He described breathing and reverse breathing[2] in great detail, laying out their physical benefits and presenting various related exercises. 'Do not underestimate the power of these few words of instruction,' he said. 'I have observed this practice every day from my youth to the present day.' The old priest, in his warm and kind manner, reiterated several critical aspects of the practice. He instructed me to

---

1 一吸便提, 息息歸臍; 一提便嚥, 水火相見 (*yi xi bian ti, xi xi gui qi; yi ti bian yan, shui huo xiang jian*): The phrase consists of 16 Chinese characters, the "Sixteen Gold Ingots" (十六錠金, *shiliu dingjin*) referred to in the title of this chapter.

2 逆式呼吸 (*nishi huxi*): A learned breathing pattern where the lower belly is actually sucked in during inhalation, and released during exhalation.

harness my full intention when inhaling, focusing it on the area of inhalation, and he showed me how to completely relax between the breaths. He pointed out that when these practices are performed for some duration, saliva will accumulate and fill the mouth, and explained how this saliva should be swallowed—he instructed me on all of these with great clarity. He also told me that when I had advanced to a higher level in my study of the Dao, I should be sure to read two books: the *Zhuangzi* and the *Yellow Court Classic*.

Although I was young then, I took these instructions to heart: several times each day, I practiced what the master had demonstrated. The oddest thing was, from the time I began this practice, the maladies that used to often peck and pester my health vanished and never reappeared. Two years later, a terrible flu was going around, and almost every member of my family contracted it. Shortly afterwards, my mother was diagnosed with a serious infectious disease, tuberculosis. At that time, tuberculosis was a global pandemic. Things seemed to be coming to pass just as the master had said, these diseases being the hazardous conditions he had alluded to. Armored with the daily meditation and exercises I had steadfastly practiced, I was able to avoid falling prey to the horrible illness. I remained immune, even as family members around me contracted the infection."

This is the sum of what Priest Tong relayed that night at the table regarding the events of his youth and his fated encounters with the old Daoist of Baiyun Temple in Shanghai.

Sifu spoke: "You must truly have sown the seeds of good fortune to have this fateful meeting at such a young age. In my own youth, I encountered a Daoist adept from Zhejiang who had studied in a lineage akin to the Dragon Gate Sect's[3] Fei Yangxi. He was quite erudite, having dipped into the great texts of Confucianism, Buddhism, and Daoism. By his account, all of his study and cultivation practices

---

3   龍門派 (*longmenpai*): Founded between the Song and Yuan dynasties, it is a branch of Wang Chongyang's School of Complete Reality, which advocates control of anger and desires, synthesis of Confucianism and Buddhism, obedience to rules and commandments, diligent practice of inner alchemy.

were based on Min Yide's (1758–1836) convenient methods of practice. He thus recommended that I consult Min's *Light of the Mind on Mt. Jindai* and *Collection of Ancient Books from the Tower of the Bookish Hermit*. Truly, in these works are a plethora of oral tips from the Dragon Gate Sect. The texts are records of Min Yide's process of devoted study, and they reveal the quintessence[4] of his wisdom. Having been fairly unoccupied at the time, I devoted time to reading them in their entirety. The remarkable thing about Min Yide is that he synthesizes the essences of Confucian, Buddhist, and Daoist doctrines, melding their complementary practices. In fact, his philosophy enables anyone with a connection to his teachings and a good heart to transform themselves. He lays out the processes of internal alchemy in great detail. For novice practitioners of that generation who had devoted their intention to entering the Dao, Min Yide's descriptions were like a guiding light.

I came to believe that Min Yide must have made a profound contribution to the School of Complete Reality. From the publication of the *Baopuzi* onward, Buddhism and Daoism had espoused distinct paths to enlightenment—Min Yide adjusted the doctrines established in antiquity. Instead of choosing a distinct path, he studied Buddhism, Daoism, and Confucianism, even Vajrayana Buddhism, melding into one the previously separate concepts of the three. He was a man of inimitable courage and insight. He was advanced in the Way, a monk of great eminence. These days as well as days past, one rarely encounters a person of such character. Furthermore, he made enormous contributions to those in subsequent generations who have sought to learn the art of the 'golden elixir.'[5] I, among them, have benefited from his work, and my admiration for him is deep. Those 'Sixteen Gold Ingots' that Mr. Tong just spoke of—I learned of them from Min Yide's successors. In fact,

---

4　玄 (*xuan*): Literally meaning a shade of black with dark red, but used in Neo-Daoist vernacular to connote the "profound."

5　丹金 (*danjin*): Authors of alchemical texts often call their tradition the "Way of the Golden Elixir" (*danjin zhi dao*). Gold (*jin*) represents immutability; Elixir (*dan*) connotes reality, principle, or true nature.

I heard the teaching several times, and the details given at each instance are fairly consistent with the account that Priest Tong has just given.

After the encounter with Min Yide's work that I just described, I appraised various ancient texts on longevity. I realized that they all mentioned the exercises derived from the 'Sixteen Gold Ingots.' Minor differences were perhaps due to the reliance on oral transmission and the many years that have passed since the original teaching: the particulars of each transmission likely had their own characteristics. Without receiving oral instruction directly from a master, there are aspects of the practice that are just beyond the grasp of a layman's sole efforts. In particular, each person's inhalation and exhalation are different, and the principles of the teaching must be adapted appropriately for each individual. Additionally, one-on-one instruction from a master to the practitioner is necessary for students to learn the proper technique for coordinating the breathing pattern with the contraction of the sphincter. Correct instruction from an experienced guide will help learners avoid any dangers of flawed practice.

Priest Tong also mentioned a few things related to Beijing Opera. According to my understanding, in the opera world there are some underground practitioners who are quite accomplished. I enjoy attending the opera and watching the performers. In the singers' technique and through the power of their voice, you can discern the depth of their skill in the Way. The strength of their foundation is evident, particularly among the martial arts performers. You have to observe their singing and actions from start to finish, see how their limbs flow through the choreography. If, amid all their leaping, bouncing, and mimes of combat, you don't hear any strain in their inhalation or exhalation, no redness in their face, no shortness of breath—this is the mark of true skill, of *gongfu*.

Back in the days I've been speaking of, there was a man called Gai Jiaotian who played warrior roles. His skill in the operatic arts was incredible. He was particularly magnificent in *Wu Song*. From beginning to end, there would never be a graceless moment in the performance. People said that Gai Jiaotian practiced breath regulation exercises every day. I heard that he could use a single inhalation for many minutes, not requiring any turn of breath, and that he had gone out of his way to learn the Daoist technique of 'turtle breathing.'

This Gai Jiaotian was rivaled in fame by one of his contemporaries, Shan Heyue, who had achieved great success in his career and was very popular; both artists performed martial arts roles. But I will tell you, there was no comparison in the quality of their performances. After a single show, Shan Heyue would clearly struggle to catch his breath. It was clear that opera performers could have many other private pursuits within their circle.

As for Gai Jiaotian, what I appreciated so much about him was not only his strong foundation in *gongfu*, but also the quality of his character, his sense of morality, and his breadth of mind. Early in his career, he was performing a sequence where there was a high risk of injuring one of his co-performers. In his attempt to prevent this, he fell upon his own leg. As soon as he fell, he knew he had broken his leg, but he summoned the strength to suppress the deep pain in his thigh. He pushed through to the curtain call, and neither the audience nor the people on stage beside him realized what had happened. Later, following leakage of the medical report that he had broken a bone, people were astonished. If someone without a foundation in *gongfu* had suffered this accident on stage, they would have passed out from the pain. How would it have been possible to maintain perfect calm and finish the show? Many people admired him for the discipline he showed in this incident.

One of the members of Gai Jiaotian's troupe once divulged that Jiaotian more than once spoke to his colleagues about another opera star, a Manchu named Tang Yunsheng, who had come to Shanghai to perform. Tang Yunsheng's abilities far outshone those of Shan Heyue; his technique was excellent. There was nothing superficial about his singing. Apparently, this Tang Yunsheng was an accomplished practitioner of the Daoist arts of cultivation. Every day he meditated and practiced breath regulation. No wonder he was so adept."

Sifu made all these remarks following Priest Tong's anecdotes. *Sifu* also offered his own interpretations of the teachings. Subsequently, all those in Daoist fellowship around the table entreated him to tell them more about the "Sixteen Gold Ingots." *Sifu* thus proceeded to outline the basics of the relevant practices, sharing with his guests what he had gained from years of study and experience: "'One inhalation facilitates rising; cycle the breath, return to the navel; one rise facilitates gulping; water and fire thus meet.' When I was young, I always practiced these exercises after meditating. The results were extraordinarily good. As I studied the words describing the practice, I realized the pricelessness of each of the 16 Chinese characters that comprise these four short phrases. When we practiced this, some would sit and some would stand. Everyone had their own way of doing it, though I will say most Daoist practitioners chose to take up a standing posture.

When preparing to do the exercise, you must first use your intention to bring relaxation throughout your body. To do so, follow the instructions I previously shared with you all: begin from your scalp, and imagine that a piece of borneol[6] is affixed to your forehead. From the crown of your head, to your forehead, continuing down through your face and all the way to the *yongquan* points on the bottom of your feet, everything must be completely relaxed. Your whole body must relax, down to each cell; this will maximize the benefits of the practice. If you are practicing directly following a sitting meditation, and *qi* is circulating throughout your body, then perform the relaxation visualization three to seven times: as you practice, adjust your breath and frame of mind until you reach a state of 'empty spirit and tranquility.' If you can obtain emptiness and stillness in your mind, then, gradually, illusions and

---

6   冰片 (*bingpian*): A medicinal substance used in Traditional Chinese Medicine, made from the sap of the camphor tree (*dryobalanops aromatica*).

negative thoughts will cease to arise. It is usually through this state that the essence of the Dao is obtained.

This method somewhat resembles what Buddhists refer to as 'resting the mind in its original place.' Generally speaking, relaxation must begin internally: in your attitude, your thinking. Then you can extend it externally throughout and over the reaches of your physical body, even into your hair and skin. Throughout your day-to-day activities, you must also strive to maintain this state of inner stillness; it is not something that should be confined to your formal practice only. Those who cultivate the Dao must be without desires or demands, without a sense of striving as they go about each day. Finally, in this manner, you will be able to enter a state of peace. Whenever you return to a meditative state, your patience will increase. The hold that everything worldly—love, lust, corruption—has on you will slowly weaken. Once avarice has been expelled, illusions and negative thoughts will naturally diminish. A practitioner may even become totally free of desire, delusive thought, and grasping. Fortunately, through training, you can cultivate this kind of temperament. This method is what Chan[7] refers to as the 'mind abiding in its place.'

If, through your practice, you are able to attain the stage whereby the mind resides in its place yet does not abide in anything, and the spirit and *qi* contain the spirit within themselves, the myriad conditions will naturally be transformed, and only the original *qi* remain. With sustained practice, remaining in a state free of nothingness and no-nothingness, your body and mind will relax deeply into a state of emptiness. If the practitioner can cultivate all pith instructions within this state of emptiness, there is nothing he or she cannot achieve.

The standing posture is the root of all posting practice: in the

---

7   禪門 (*chanmen*): Chan (Zen, as it is commonly known in its Japanese form) Buddhism, one of the main sects of the Mahayana Buddhist tradition, whose first patriarch was the legendary Bodhidharma (達摩), who traveled from the Indian subcontinent to China, consequently spreading the Buddha's teachings throughout North and East Asia.

Daoist school and on the path of immortality, it must be practiced regularly. During standing practice, it is best to stand with your face toward the eastern sunlight. After your body has relaxed, according to the aforementioned methods, sink slightly into your stance, with the feet spaced shoulder-width apart. Completely align your vertebrae and relax your sacral region. Direct your focus toward the inside of your mouth and around your tongue, using your tongue to swirl your saliva. When saliva has completely filled your mouth, begin coordinating with your inhalations; fix your whole mind in one place, focusing only on the *qi*. Simultaneously, gurgle and swallow your saliva, and use your intention to slightly contract your anus. While doing so, bring your *qi* to cover your *dantian*;[8] that is, you should unite the *qi* from the upper half of your body and that from the lower half of your body at the [lower] *dantian*. After the *qi* from the upper and lower regions have met in the *dantian*, pause and focus on your navel. Using your inhaled *qi*, put pressure on the *dantian* from above and below. As if practicing 'precious vase *qigong*,'[9] hold your breath. The power and speed of the practice should match your level of expertise in it. Just note that when you squeeze your anus, you shouldn't use too much force, otherwise you may induce hemorrhoids. When you expel the *qi*, relax your anus. At the point of relaxation, some Daoist practitioners manipulate the vital energy from the aforementioned section of the *dantian*, moving the *qi* into the governing channel.[10] That is, they bring the energy up from the sacrum and into the crown of the head as they forcefully exhale.

Before receiving the teaching of the 'Sixteen Gold Ingots,' practitioners should have a foundation in posting. If they have not

---

8   丹田 (*dantian*): Literally, "red field" or "cinnabar field." It is a focal point and energy center for most *qigong* and meditation practices, located approximately four finger widths below the navel, inside the lower abdomen.

9   寶瓶氣功 (*baoping qigong*): A preliminary practice in Vajrayana Buddhism preparing the yogi for more advanced teachings.

10   督脈 (*dumai*): The "Sea of Yang Meridians" which "governs" and is the convergence of all the *yang* channels in the body. It flows up the midline of the back, from the tailbone to the top of the head and then drops down to the roof of the mouth.

yet established this foundation, then it is best that they first study posting and later receive the teaching through oral transmission. The importance of the Daoist posting practice should not be underestimated. I can testify that the late Wang Xiangzhai (1885–1963) was a master of this practice. Taking one breath, standing in place, he could be surrounded by ten people, all pushing on his body from different sides, and he wouldn't waver: this evinces *gongfu*. When you practice posting, you should gradually transfer your whole body's center of gravity to the *yongquan* points. Along with your weight, the *qi* also pours into the *yongquan*. As the *qi* passes through the *dantian* downward, summon it back up from the 'bubbling wells,' passing it through the 'three gates,'[11] and finally bringing it to the upper *dantian* (*niwan*) at the crown of the head. Then bring it back down to the *yongquan*, completing one breath cycle: that is, absorb more *qi*, release less. This method leads to truly incredible results."

---

11 三關 (*sanguan*): Three points along the governing channel that are frequently obstructed, these are in the area of the tailbone, opposite the center of the chest and the back of the head.

CHAPTER 3

SINCERE AND BLAMELESS— STILL THE MIND AND BECOME A SAGE

Sifu continued: "Now, just yesterday I was talking with several disciples who had completed the microcosmic orbit.[1] Generally speaking, my teaching on meditation diverges slightly from the traditional teachings. After arriving in Taiwan, I made minor adjustments to my teaching in accordance with the lifestyles of people here. It is terribly difficult to convince a modern person to dedicate one or two hours each day to meditation. Additionally, if one is to teach this effectively, the use and origins of the practice must first be clearly explained. My personal view is that the most critical aspect of meditation is not how long one sits, how long one can keep one's vertebrae aligned, how long your back stays straight—these are all physical skills. To build up physical stamina, all you need is endurance, time, and will. What fewer and fewer people pay attention to is that the most important aspect of meditation is your state of mind.

Growing up under the influence of a scholarly family, I had begun reading the great works of the sages and of Confucianism before studying the Dao. My father especially stressed the Confucian school of idealist philosophy from the Song and Ming dynasties. As a child, I was required to master the schools of thought and philosophical lineages of Cheng Hao and Cheng Yi; my father was deeply knowledgeable of both. From the Wei, Jin, Northern,

---

1   小周天 (*xiaozhoutian*): Daoist practices that involve moving the *qi* through channels in an elliptical "orbit" around the body.

and Southern Dynasties (220–589), the arrival and dissemination of Buddhism in China, through the Confucian schools of the Song Dynasty and how they intersected with the essential teachings of Buddhism to inform the classical studies of the Song and Ming era literati, all of these relationships he knew like the back of his hand.

From early on, my family also engaged the services of a certain Master Zhang, a talented scholar and county-level imperial official during the final years of the Qing Dynasty. My cousins and I studied with this master, whom, back then, we referred to simply as 'Sir.' He was highly learned: in addition to Confucian scholarship, he was well versed in countless literary works spanning the four forms of Chinese poetry. Often, during a period of silence, Master Zhang would knowingly nod his head and begin to chant a poem. He would simultaneously demonstrate techniques for memorizing poetry and impart upon us each poem's context and related anecdotes. His methods of instruction ensured that the content of the great poetic works were deeply impressed upon each of the pupils; we would be hard pressed to forget. The central theme of his lectures was the principle of benevolence, and instruction on personal disposition was the basis of his teachings; the system of thought attributed to Ming Dynasty scholar Liu Zongzhou (1578–1645) was the root of his philosophy. Ancestors of this Master Zhang had studied under Liu Zongzhou in the Classical Academy, so his home had been filled with the written works of the latter: Sir had thus been steeped in an environment of scholarship and conservation practices from a young age. Sincerity and propriety were woven into the very core of his being. He often instructed us: a true gentleman must observe strict self-discipline every day as he goes about his business; he must never assume that he can abandon principle in private life just because no one is watching or no one is aware of his behavior; his disposition must always remain consistent with principle, otherwise he may manifest improper behaviors. Over time, everyone will come to recognize and respect him for his consistent uprightness in disposition and behavior. The meaning of 'sincerity' is nothing more than not deceiving oneself. Those on the path of study must unify the internal and external worlds; desires must be controlled in all things. Whether one is moving, dwelling, sitting or lying down, one's sense of right and wrong must clearly be at the forefront at all times.

Throughout the speeches and silences, the activity and stillness of his daily life, Master Zhang's eyes never seemed entirely open, lids perpetually hung half-closed. I suspect this state had something to do with the fact that he never passed a day without meditating.

Master Zhang would often recite the inherited teachings of Zhu Xi [also known as Zhuzi, a Confucian writer, 1130–1200] on methods of meditation for our class of boys: according to our teacher, Zhu Xi held himself to a rigorous schedule of practice—he would spend half of each day with a quiet mind in sitting meditation. Deeply influenced by Zhu Xi's example, the later philosopher Wang Yangming (1472–1529) also observed a strict routine of daily meditation.

From the time I was a young child, then, I studied Confucian theory and doctrine with Master Zhang, gaining considerably from these many years under his tutelage. He was the first meditation teacher I encountered who was an enlightened master. When he taught about the art of meditation, he would not emphasize the cross-legged posture; rather he taught us to sit in a chair, with our feet touching the floor, back straight, vertebrae relaxed and gently pulling away from each other, top to bottom, in alignment. He instructed us to hold the head straight like a brush poised for calligraphy, slightly draw in the lower jaw, fix the eyes on a point in front of us, and let the face soften into a contented expression. He emphasized the principles of respect and seeking truth at the root, and taught us that after these had been thoroughly assimilated, the examination of one's temperament should meld into the focus of meditation. The result would be something similar to the Chan practice of resting the mind in its original place.

Sometime later, I read some of Zhu Xi's essays and notes on these matters. In his discussion, he often mentions that when practicing martial arts, one must first set up a guard over, and come to an understanding of, the mind. He also illuminates the appropriate starting point for those just beginning the pursuit of the Way. Zhu Xi is unusual among the great Confucian scholars in the considerable efforts he devoted to the study of Buddhist and Daoist meditation practices. In fact, among the multitude of Confucian scholars, he is the only one to frequently admonish students to meditate more, warning that otherwise they would certainly stray from the straight path.

Generally speaking, across Confucianism, Buddhism, and Daoism, 'stillness' is emphasized as the critical starting point for unifying the body, mind, and spirit. *The Great Learning* also underscores that only by first achieving stillness can one deepen into stability. If the mind is not still, the *qi* and the spirit will inevitably be slack. A person who maintains a disposition of stillness long-term will exhibit vastly greater concentration than others. Nothing in the environment of such a practitioner will disturb them. From this state, one can reach a plane of desirelessness, shedding all irrationality, pensiveness, and pursuits. Finally, of course, one can attain a state of being which is not disturbed by a single particle of worldly pollution: not a single thought arises, and the inner and outer worlds have become empty through and through. Thus, considering the potential of their guidance, I have deep respect for the meditation teachings of the great Confucian scholars.

It is said that the learned scholar Liu Zhitang (1767–1855), of the late Qing era, nearly died when he was a young man, but he encountered a talented teacher who transmitted to him teachings related to the art of achieving stillness. Essentially, once Liu had understood how to quiet his mind, he was able to rescue his body from the brink of danger and achieve a state of peace and stability, even transcendence. Thereafter, because of this fortuitous encounter, Liu Zhitang instructed all of his followers to meditate daily. He taught that daily meditation would enable them to nourish virtue and strengthen the body. In all of Sichuan, there was no one who did not respect and esteem the great Confucian master Liu.

The methods I am describing belong to the Daoist tradition. However, I have always maintained that if a technique only allows movement through the macrocosmic and microcosmic orbit practices but does not facilitate understanding of the cultivation of mental calm and a fundamental outlook based on the principle of a quieted mind, then at best, after practicing such a technique, one will not differ much from an average person, with perhaps only slightly less focus on worldly habits. But if one pairs the cultivation of stillness with breathing practices, regulation in inhalation and exhalation, then over time one's mind will naturally calm and sink into limpid stillness. The spirit and *qi* will become self-sufficient, and the seven emotions will be short-lived; progressing one step further, one may awake to the reality of emptiness. The practitioner will understand emptiness, and will enter the state where one is empty even of emptiness. Accordingly, before I agree to train a student in Daoist breathing exercises, I always first assess whether he has a foundation in stillness. If he lacks this foundation, he must first build it up for at least half a year. His vulnerability to lustful passions and covetousness must be diminished, and his delusions and attachments must melt away. Only then can he manifest clear results from Daoist instruction."

The preceding account comprises all that the master shared with all present—the elders and younger folks and all those in Daoist fellowship—at the banquet I mentioned. In response to the questions and discussion of that evening's guests, he described these matters regarding how to reach higher levels of stillness and perfection in sitting meditation.

CHAPTER 4

How to Cultivate Vast *Qi* amidst Fame and Fortune

Let us address how a beginner should approach sitting meditation and entering stillness. Unlike the ancients, the modern person has no way to establish a space for stillness in their home or anywhere else. Therefore, the only way for people in this day and age to access a place of true meditative stillness in their daily activities is through the regulation of the breath, the careful practice of inhalation and exhalation. Many people experience great suffering amidst the noise and perplexity of this world: the manifold sources of worldly pollution can bring about negative internal states and a depressed frame of mind. In some people whose existence is joyless and prone to depression long term, the four elements will stop regulating each other properly, and the five internal organ systems will become unbalanced. This can lead to clinical depression, anxiety disorders, insomnia, nervous breakdowns, cardiovascular diseases, illnesses of the digestive system, ulcers, all manner of gynecological diseases, and other health problems. All of these maladies come about when one does not understand the importance of relieving the mind and regulating the breath: the condition known in Chinese Medicine as "vacuous heat rising in the body"[1] will arise. This makes one vulnerable to inflammation, and if this state is left unchecked over time, the roots of infection will begin to take hold in all of the body's cells. The plague of this era, cancer, is indeed connected to psychological vulnerabilities—60 percent of cases have roots and are triggered by a dis-ease of the mind. In humans,

---

1   虚火上升 (*xu huo shang sheng*): In Traditional Chinese Medicine, a condition in which heat rises in the body due to vacuity (also translated as "deficiency").

diseases emerging from the body–mind relationship are not merely a phenomenon of the modern age: ever since the creation of the cosmos, the *qi* that connects people to heaven and earth and facilitates their movement through the world has depended on their daily breathing. Thus, if one cannot grasp the proper methods of inhalation and exhalation, or the techniques of breath regulation, illness is naturally unavoidable.

The key to breathing exists within the mind: it is dictated by the regulated inhalations and exhalations and is best cultivated amid the three interrelated vital treasures—*qi*, essence, and spirit. Internal *qi* manifests in the seven emotions and six desires: if a person regularly experiences excessive worry, and vexation has a firm hold within them, a surplus of emotions—from happiness to grief—will flow out of them. Their internal clock will be a mess, with their circadian rhythm and sleep–wake cycle misaligned; they will also be prone to debauchery and will not know how to control themselves; they will be smug but without satisfaction; under the long-term influence of unhappy, grievous, or violent *qi*, internal fire will rise and become difficult to quell. And all of these consequences are due to not understanding how to nourish *qi*, regulate breath, store the spirit. Without this understanding, one's premature demise is nearly certain; longevity is almost impossible to obtain.

As Daoist immortals[2] of lore were wont to say, "the cultivation of *qi* through breathing exercises is the medicine for 100 years." For one's temperament to contribute to longevity, one must cultivate *qi*, essence, and spirit in concert, and *qi* is the key to the connection and flow among them. Thus, as stated above, many people who practiced Daoism in ages past emphasized the dual cultivation of body and mind, and to this they would add the Confucian disciplines of *qi* cultivation and right conduct. Among these practices, the most effective and widely known is the method Mencius

---

2   真人 (*zhenren*): "Immortality" in the Daoist sense does not imply eternal life, but rather signifies the highest achievement in the Daoist practice, which also carries with it an extended life span.

described for cultivating *qi*—this was the mainstream method of cultivation in the Confucian school during the Song-Ming era.

If a person understands how to regulate and cultivate *qi*, their whole body will be in harmony, with the systems functioning smoothly; thus, they will naturally exude awe-inspiring righteousness. Over time, they may reach a state of harmony with nature and the heavens. The gains from meditation and breath regulation are the protection and nourishment of *qi*. If *qi* is muddled, spirit will be scattered, essence will be lost, one's true spirit will depart, and it will be hard to preserve the soul. One may sit quietly for 100 years, resulting in nothing: if the sitting is meditation in name only, the final result will certainly be a pointless death.

The origin point of true *qi* lies in the location where breath enters and leaves in the correct practice of continuous, smooth respiration. Daoist masters of ages past all acknowledged this point and its importance to opening the mind. From start to finish, the mind must maintain flexible and expansive discernment. One must not be attached to the ephemeral allures of the external world; the beauty of a song is as fleeting as flowing water. To someone who understands these matters, a dangerous tsunami that reaches the sky is no great matter. With this level of *qi* cultivation and breadth of mind, the drawing in and expulsion of breath is extraordinary, as are all aspects of the cultivation and results of the practice.

These are all principles that I encountered in my youth after I had completed the initial parts of my education in meditation at *sifu*'s residence. The importance of the mind was central to his instruction. He often remarked that the traditional jargon from the ancient Daoist teachings must be translated into terms that modern people can receive—only then will the messages be useful to the world. We should not cling to old formalisms, without the courage to challenge orthodoxy, muddying the lines between what's credible and what's not. If you seem to call the same thing a cauldron and then a stove, a dragon and then a tiger, water and then fire, what is a modern person to make of it? They won't know right from wrong. They will see the teacher as lofty and far-removed from them, and will be scared to pursue the path of study. This in fact equates to sowing the karmic seeds of slander of the true Path. *Sifu* often said that people in this day and age need not add yet more focus to the matters of mortal flesh; those involved in business, those rolling about in fame and fortune, should be shown how to see through and eventually let go of the Eight Worldly Winds.[3] Thereafter, they will be able to complete the microcosmic orbit without hindrance. If a person reaches a clear understanding of Heaven and Earth and everything in between, and can transcend any consideration of the bounds of life and death, then they will have also realized the macrocosmic orbit.[4]

The life of Su Dongpo is the greatest example of these teachings. At times his life was a constant roll in worldly affairs; at times glory and failure met in opposition on this path, as did both fortune and devastation. He was destitute in cold and sweltering landscapes; he sunk into entanglements with no means for changing his fate; at times he was lionized but had no outlet for showing his exhaustion. He had a lofty reputation for his talents and achievements, but he sometimes encountered difficulties as a scholar. As a member of the literati, he spent his whole life on the precarious path of the learned, each day spent in a bundle of anxiety. And though he sometimes dwelt on studying and indulging in mountain scenery, he couldn't hold at bay the contradictions in his heart. Sometimes he wanted to mold himself to uprightness, but again, a lesser nature would overtake him and he would not be able to suppress vile impulses. Later on, he had a couple of curious encounters, but one after the other these situations ended in disaster. Truly, it was only by living a lifestyle beyond the pale of civilization that Su Dongpo began to understand the reality of monks' teachings. Thus, although he

---

3   世俗八法 (*shi su ba fa*): The winds of activity and change that can knock us off our feet. These include the complementary opposites of gain and loss, pleasure and pain, praise and blame, and fame and shame.
4   大周天 (*dazhoutian*): An extension of the "microcosmic orbit" practice incorporating the arms and legs.

never became a master of martial arts or enlightenment in the highest sense, he did achieve a profound understanding of the practice of health cultivation and meditation, and his perspective on these matters was unique. Detailed study of Su Dongpo's canon reveals his early fated connection with Chan Buddhism and Daoism: as a young man he had already won the favor of the famous Daoist priest Zhang Yijia—the priest singled out Su Dongpo from 100 students to receive his teachings.

Su Dongpo's schoolmate Chen Taichu was also a person of great stature. In later years, Chen did not accrue the same degree of fame as Su Dongpo, but he did devote himself to the cultivation of the Dao. The final act he is known for is his incredible feat of liberating his soul from his body and appearing as an immortal to later generations. This anecdote is recorded in the major histories; everyone has heard of these events. It is said that Priest Chen passed away while sitting cross-legged in meditation. Upon finding him, the chief of the prefecture, unaware of the lofty identity attached to the body he had discovered, ordered the corpse be disposed of on the outskirts of the city among the wild weeds and thistles. The young soldier who received this order felt ill at ease, and as he was carrying the body complained the whole way, "How unlucky! This is terribly inauspicious that I've been commanded to carry a dead Daoist priest during the height of major New Year's festivities!" And the whole time the young fellow was walking and crying out about his miserable fate, he didn't realize that Chen Taichu had come back to life. In fact, Chen had gotten up and walked off, passing under a bridge, beside which he sat down to meditate. From there, he simply got up and departed this world. All of the people in the area came to know of this marvel. But, truly, there have been so many of this sort of fantastic event in the history of Daoism that they can hardly be considered extraordinary.

In his day-to-day life, whenever Su Dongpo had free time, he would spend it meditating. He knew that this classmate of his had connected with the Dao and reached the stage of moving the celestial chariot[5] early in life. Su Dongpo deeply envied and admired his friend for this, and he also understood that, in his own life, it would be extremely difficult for him to transcend his fame and wealth to reach a similar point. He knew that to cultivate the Dao and attain authenticity is impossible without otherworldly resolve and rigorous examination and understanding. It is as the ancient sages said: the so-called "immortal" is a virtuous person without dreams. After his awakening, he has no worries. His food is light and tasteless. Only his breathing is deep. To him, there is no boundary between living and dying. He comes and goes as he pleases, is not manipulated by anything, and is at ease always. He has no demands toward his final destiny, but he does not forget the genesis of his life. He doesn't care about favors or humiliations. His mind does not grasp at the Dao, and his method does not grasp at his mind. The immortal's *gongfu* is not affected by the changing seasons, by the common vicissitudes of human life. Directly in the way of flowing water, he will not be weakened; walking into fire, he will not burn; ascending to great heights, he will not fear. And his fasts will help his digestion.

---

5   河車搬運 (*he che ban yun*): A practice of circulating *qi* through the governing and conception channels.

CHAPTER 5

Unmoved by the Eight Winds—The Nature of Mental Cultivation

Outside of his deep exploration of Daoism and Chan, Su Dongpo's days were fraught, and he faced complications and dangers on his path as an official statesman. These experiences engendered in him an earnest appreciation of his life and health. He often exhorted his family members and disciples: right and wrong, glory and dishonor must not be mixed up together in your dealings; when you encounter a problem, it shouldn't derail all other aspects of your life; when difficulties come your way, you should consider them as if they were playing out in a stage performance—don't take anything too seriously; at no time, under no circumstance, should you let thorns take root in your heart—pull them out; without hesitation, deftly cut all the common worldly bitternesses out of your life; regularly consider your worldly attachments—besides your thoughts and your physical body, you have nothing; all worldly possessions are illusions—how much more illusory are the swirling thoughts of your mind; the foundation of composed conduct in society is deep and careful thinking; in your behavior, it is important to deal with things unhurriedly; the only way to avoid base people is to refrain from being greedy; modesty, reserve, and being accepting and forgiving are the skills needed to preserve harmonious relations; when you have the right person for a job, you should support them emotionally by being forgiving and reserved; to adjust your thinking and deportment to suit all situations and people is an art natural to refined people.

Su Dongpo often advised those near him to sleep well, eat well, and exert themselves in physical labor and exercise. For worldly people, emptying the mind of substance is a marvelous attainment. When he encountered people with whom he shared a sense of karmic destiny, he did not hesitate to transmit to them the longevity-cultivating Daoist breathing exercises he had learned from his personal studies of Daoism: the Daoist *baduanjin*,[1] the "12-Step Brocade for Cultivating Longevity through [Qi] Bathing,"[2] the whole-body practice of the five-element-based movements, etc., all techniques that Su Dongpo used personally to cultivate good health and long life. He often said that, even though he spent much time meditating, he believed that more important than one's state in sitting meditation is the temperament one displays following seated practice.

In one particular instance, after he had emerged from meditation, a poem appeared in his mind. He wrote it down, and it is widely known among all who have come after him:

I bow my head to the heaven within heaven
Hairline rays illuminating the universe
The eight winds cannot move me
Sitting still upon the purple golden lotus

Originally, "I bow my head to the heaven within heaven" was a line of poetry used in rituals of worship before the Buddhas of the Ten Directions, and also to describe the Buddha's stately and auspicious expression. However, in the middle of the poem is a reference to the author's relationship to worldly matters: "The eight winds cannot move me." The line is somewhat contentious and smug in tone. The realm beyond the eighth Bodhisattva plane is well devoid of all differentiation between self and other, so what use is there then of any

---

1 八段錦: Also known as "Eight Pieces of Brocade" or "Eight Silken Movements." A set of *qigong daoyin* exercises for boosting health, it is also used as a form of martial arts training. It is discussed at length in Chapter 25, and the second half of the Practice Guide and Exercises in Part 2 offers detailed instructions for practice.

2 十二長生沐浴導引術 (*shier changsheng muyu daoyin shu*): "Bathing" here does not involve water but a series of patting, rubbing, and other vigorous movement exercises that a practitioner might use first thing in the morning to wake up the body and move the *qi*. Discussed in Chapter 17, the first half of the Practice Guide and Exercises in Part 2 offers a manual for its practice.

of the eight winds of fame and gain, honor and disrepute, praise and blame, or happiness and suffering? This line clearly demonstrates that Su Dongpo had not yet reached enlightenment—he was overly complacent. At that time, he had been demoted, but it was not the first bump in his official career, and he had become numb to such misfortunes; so, it was nearly inevitable that he would write in such a self-mocking way. Additionally, he was quite pleased with himself that in those days he had been able to use the methods of meditation to discipline and purify his mind of vexations. Thus, he penned this line. But he knew that this couldn't fool his close friend Master Foyin, who lived outside of regular Chinese society. Upon hearing the poem, Master Foyin indeed made a tongue-in-cheek amendment to the last line, ridiculing Su Dongpo:

The eight winds cannot move me
One fart blows me across the river

The reaction Su Dongpo had to Master Foyin's response to his poem is not the main point here: the point is that this exchange exemplifies what happens to so many people with slackened resolve in states of arrogance, poverty, or other straits, who lack an enlightened teacher as well as the means of dissolving the self-loathing and endless worry in their hearts. Sometimes this results in people losing their very lives: they have no way to carry on. On that topic, when I was studying at *sifu*'s residence, I heard certain stories from one of the old Daoist priests I was familiar with. This deeply warm and peaceful man was highly practiced in the Daoist cultivation arts. In his early years, he had lived and studied at sacred temples in places such as the Yandang Mountains and on Mount Lao. He had met many advanced practitioners. Thus, before he had even turned 30, he had already totally cleared his conception and governing channels.[3] My first time encountering this elder, I

---

3   任督二脈 (*ren du er mai*): Two energy channels in the body that play a primary role in *qigong* practice and together form the microcosmic orbit: the *ren* vessel runs through the center of the ventral portion of the body; the *du* channel runs through the center of the dorsal portion of the body.

envied his extraordinary and effortless grace. From the age of 60 onward, he had let his beard and mustache grow long, and he wore a long navy robe. He was debonair in his bearing. After that first encounter, I did have some contact with him, but he encountered an unfortunate event that everyone in the Daoist circles considered a pity: an old acquaintance from his village arranged for him to be married to a newly widowed woman to help him with household chores and be a companion to him.

Unexpectedly, less than one year after the marriage, the elderly Daoist's new wife bundled up his life savings and valuables and disappeared, sending no messages thereafter. The man never recovered from this blow, and even developed amnesia. Thus, it can be seen that the crux of Daoist practices is cultivation of one's disposition, and that on this path of Daoist cultivation one is sure to encounter innumerable obstacles and checkpoints. It is not an easy road. For this reason, *sifu*, in his great wisdom and far-sightedness, began advising me early on and often in my practice that to meditate poorly, to sit in boredom as if a plant, to hold the shape of an expanse of stagnant water, to become still like a corpse, is to waste one's existence, to have come into the earth and inhabited a body pointlessly.

Because of the ever-rising fortune of the days of my youth, I encountered good teachers who transmitted to me the true path to wisdom. Thus, after many years under the encouragement of *sifu*, I had read the Confucian classics as well as the quintessential books of the Daoist canon. And the most important teachings I received were in how to establish and comport oneself in society, how to be worldly wise—these were of enormous benefit to me.

CHAPTER 6

ASSESS ONESELF— CONSERVE THE MIND, RETURN TO STILLNESS

My aim here is not, in fact, to suggest that modern people must follow the path of the ancients, nor to say they must sit like a statue in lotus position. I am not even prescribing that people meditate for a certain number of hours every day. The main thing when beginning a sitting meditation practice is to adjust one's mind and breathing, so that *qi* and mind can become one. The emphasis of meditation is therefore on how to breathe. Just because the word "sitting" is in "sitting meditation" does not mean one should focus on the physical act of sitting down. To truly "sit," one must first experience in the physical being a state of mind that is peaceful, limpid, far removed from the madding crowds, wholly free from the world's pollution, spotless. Whether in walking, dwelling, sitting, or lying down, one's intuitive consciousness must be preserved, and one must be unfettered in one's ability to access and control breathing at all times. Then, when one enters sitting meditation, one can at any moment take on the state of "unifying breath and mind."[1] This is the best meditation method for most people in this day and age. If your goal is to become a cultivator of *qi*, though, you must also be intimately acquainted with all of the classical texts on Daoist cultivation practices. Additionally, at some point in your life, you must spend three years far removed from the polluted world. You must seal yourself in quiet for this period, and you must

---

1   心息一處 (*xin xi yi chu*): When the mind and the breath are unified, they can be placed at and focused upon certain points (e.g., on the tip of the nose).

be under the guidance of an enlightened, experienced teacher. This is the only way to give yourself the chance to experience what those in the Daoist school allude to as "another realm."

Some modern people may have already experienced the afore-mentioned breath regulation practices. Those who, thereafter, desire to move deeper into understanding, should focus on the hard work of cultivating the temperament through internal prac-tice. In general, it is recommended every day, after awakening, to first firmly seize whatever shadowy traces of thought linger for a moment; then, let go of every doubt and hindrance from yesterday. Remind yourself that in this new day, you will encounter a different realm, and that you will need a positive, progressive bearing to face what lies ahead. Rumination must be reduced to the smallest possible scope. You should avoid all sensory things of the outer realm that tempt you to stray from the right path. When you walk, focus all your attention on your lower *dantian*, about three or four finger-widths below your navel. The *dantian* is the focal point for conserving and absorbing *qi* and cultivating your body and mind.

If you have time, you should meditate. If the time for medita-tion is short, it is sufficient to train your mind on the quintessential Confucian principle of *jing*.[2] Your head must sit perfectly upright; avoid crookedness. Your eyes should look out level, directly in front of you, and be fixed on a point. Both feet should be flat on the floor, with the whole foot touching the earth, like the feet of a goose. Your hands should be slightly cupped, one on top of the other, the hollow of your palms facing downward, placed on your lap, below the navel. Your mouth is like a sealed scar over a wound. The focus of your entire body should be on breath regulation: deflect all exterior stimuli and suspend your thoughts, attend to the breath single-mindedly. This is the starting point that the great Confucian sages referred to as "single-minded focus on proper bearing, unfettered by external disturbances."

If your mind can be at ease like a homebody, and is hidden

---

2 敬: "Propriety," (i.e., things being how/where they ought to be).

from the vastness of the outside world, focusing only on dwelling within the home, then that space becomes the whole world. Therefore, in such an expanse of space, gather your mind and relax your body–mind; gather your thoughts and confirm that nothing in them violates Heaven's laws. Take care to note whether you have any public or private matters that hint at a tendency toward deception. Nothing should arise that diminishes your virtue and is harmful to humanity. As you move through your daily life, do not engage in any unethical behavior. Having completed your work for the day, if you have some free time, you should take a moment to examine yourself and your consciousness to see if some of the aforementioned ills are present. If so, you must immediately reflect on your mind. This is the skill Confucians refer to as "calling oneself to one's senses." Sages like Zhu Xi used to contextualize all their philosophical inquiries within the prosaic happenings of daily life. After you read the sage's accounts, rest and meditate, adjusting your mind and breath; over time, your mind will become peaceful and your *qi* will stabilize. Everything will be illuminated; aspects of the Dao that were previously difficult to understand will naturally come into clarity and focus.

If one persists in this practice of meditation and attention to one's mind, a unity of mind around the Dao will become accessible. The sort of single-mindedness I am speaking of is the pure, foundational mental state of every individual. The foremost teaching of Zhu Xi and other major Confucian figures was that people should prioritize benevolence above all, and should not give up paying attention to their mind: cultivation efforts should be focused on the mind, and one should meditate to enable the principle of *jing* to be foremost in one's consciousness. Gradually, you will also be able to achieve stillness while moving about—that is, there will be no state in which you are not attuned to meditative stillness. Whether in moving about, at home, in sitting or lying down, whether in leisure or labor, all states will be characterized by the principle of the Dao.

Meditation is the ultimate fixing of attention. When most people get a moment of mental peace, it may be difficult to prevent the mind from straying toward external things. The mind in this instance is like a house pet: when released, its heart will turn to the outside world, and eventually it will forget to return to its home. In this regard, Confucian meditation practice differs from that of Buddhism or Daoism. Confucian meditation practice does not emphasize attaining enlightenment through seeing one's self-nature or ascending to the heavens an immortal. Rather, one must simply have control of one's mind, being able to gather and send it out to fixed points. This ability is what Mencius was referring to when he said:

> Benevolence is man's mind, and righteousness is man's path. How lamentable is it to neglect the path and not pursue it, to lose this mind and not know to seek it again! When men's fowls and dogs are lost, they know to seek for them again, but they lose their mind, and do not know to seek for it. The great end of learning is nothing else but to seek for the lost mind.[3]

Everyone has a foundational mental state, and to "place the mind," as it were, is to retrieve that foundational attention that has been lost, that has departed from the person. In day-to-day life, the average person will easily let the direction of their mind slip as they encounter the circumstances of the outside world. They are reluctant to part with material treasures, sensual pleasures, and empty matters of reputation and fame. Thus, they lose their mental clarity and exhaust their bodies. Gradually, the mind is overwhelmed with emotions and desires, giving rise to various disorders of the mind and the nervous system. The individual's original ideals and sense of direction will be worn down to nothing.

The way to guard one's temperament is just as Confucius described in the *Xiao Min* ("Heavens") chapter of the *Xiao Ya* ("Lesser Court Hymns") section of the *Classic of Poetry*. Although this passage was originally directed toward individuals of great

---

3   Translated by James Legge, quoted in the Chinese Text Project, https://ctext.org/mengzi/gaozi-i.

power and status in the imperial court, it is still pertinent to ordinary people who are seeking to act humanely in society. When doing one's utmost to take care and act prudently, one should be continuously alert to one's state of mind. As soon as one's attention to the matters of the mind slips, so too will one's mind; it will spiral into the void. This is akin to the ever-present possibility of death. It is as if one is standing on an extremely thin sheet of ice—if one's attention slips and one takes too heavy a step, balance will be lost and the one treading on ice will fall through. The danger here is real, and this is the reason we meditate. The core intention is to edify the mind and prevent it from deviating from the correct path.

Thus, Daoism and Confucianism differ from Buddhism in meditative states and in the main emphases of meditation practice; however, this is most evident with Chan, whose view is even more ultimate. Someone once asked a Chan teacher: "What is meditative stillness?" The teacher replied: "When no delusive thoughts arise, this is meditation. When the sitter realizes their original nature, this is stillness." The "original nature" referred to here, and the "foundational mind" referred to by Zhu Xi are not exactly the same thing. "Original nature" refers to our inner mind being immovable, our original face beyond birth and death. It is absolutely clear, without fabrication, ungraspable and unshakable. So-called "concentration," is to be blind and deaf to the myriad stimulations of the outside world. A person with concentration is as if made from wood: no thoughts alight on their environment, their mental activity is unmoved by it. They have arrived at the state in which they cannot be moved by the Eight Worldly Winds.

Someone also asked the Chan master: "How does one calm the mind to the point of abiding?" The teacher replied: "Abiding in a place of non-abiding is true abiding." Here, the meaning behind "abiding in a place of non-abiding" is that the mind cannot be attached to the differentiations, to demarcations of good and bad; this is the optimal abode for the mind. And another question: "If I may, with what sort of mind does the teacher cultivate the Dao on a day-to-day basis?" The Chan teacher replied: "This old practitioner has no mind to apply, no means for cultivation." The questioner pressed further: "If the teacher has no mind and no strategy for cultivation, then what does the teacher want with lecturing so many people about Buddhist sutras every day?" The teacher replied: "Not even the place where I am standing exists; how could there be a place to accommodate 'many people'? Furthermore, I was born without a tongue. How could I ever expound upon the Way?" The inner state revealed by this master illustrates the difference between the realms of Daoism and Chan Buddhism.

Now, let us examine the essential teachings Mencius described. His main point in this matter is actually simple, easily understood, and pertinent to modern people. In fact, it is a great help to those with body–mind fatigue, those long dwelling in the noisiness of the world. All that is needed is the ability to take hold of the original mind that's lost, the mind running amok like a wild horse. Grasp it, and turn your internal light upon it. Do not let it continue roaming aimlessly for an extended period of time. In fact, this is a precious teaching in the art of storing and releasing one's mind. When meditating, pay extra attention to changes in your emotional state. As you examine, consider this: before happiness arises, before anger arises, before sorrow arises, before joy arises, where is your still mind abiding? At noon, take advantage of any midday break you may have, and find a quiet space to sit in meditation. From the first moment you opened your eyes in the early morning to midday, have you been affected by any disorderly matter of human affairs or the external world? Has there been any period of mental abandonment, of your mind being lost and scattered among external matters? In the evening, sit yet again in meditation. Relax your body and mind, and adjust your breath. Return to the method you used at midday. If you continue to move through your days in this way, over time you will naturally obtain the wonders of a calm mind and regulated spirit.

The main purpose of the aforementioned practice of breath regulation is to calm and focus the mind. The more tranquil the mind, the more stable the person. Such a person's breathing does not require special focus, for it will naturally revert to being soft and fine for prolonged spans. In Daoism, this is where you find true breath. This is also the most profound phenomenon in inhalation and exhalation: the longer the breath cycle, the more it moves the practitioner toward achieving a cohesive state of mind and *qi*. Furthermore, the unification of mind and *qi* accords with the main focuses of the "Sixteen Gold Ingots," which we discussed at the beginning. To have all breaths return to the navel, one must know that the place to which the breath "returns" is the original source of life. Someone who is naturally inclined to this practice and can take hold of the core of this teaching may enter "fetal breathing."[4] Like the mythical tortoise of long life, they will experience the longevity of the gods.

---

4   胎息 (*taixi*): A method of Daoist breathing that involves breathing directly from the lower *dantian* without the need for air to pass into the lungs.

CHAPTER 7

STABILIZE THE MIND, CULTIVATE VITAL ENERGY

Daoism, Confucianism, any religion, any sect, any school will espouse methods of meditation, and for all of these, the starting point is always a peaceful mind. This matter I have discussed in preceding sections regarding why it is important to prioritize stillness: the principle is related to the *taiji*[1] referenced in the *Yi Jing* (*Book of Changes*). When a person's mind has reached ultimate tranquility, their kidney *qi* will naturally become more abundant and vigorous, at which point true *yang qi*[2] will be generated. This is the first step in *gongfu* when one begins a meditation practice. The technical phrase for this step is "*yi yang lai fu*."[3] It has also been called "true fire." If one continues onward in meditation practice, all of one's vital organs as well as one's *qi* and blood circulation will reach peak health, and one's immune system will be strong. When meditating, one must deflect all influence from the outside world, as much as possible. Become absorbed in inhalation and exhalation, rest the mind in its original place. If you can achieve a unified mind, the next step is for the body to be full of the positive force of true *qi*: the mind will be totally void of any worries or hindrances. At this point, one will experience the phenomenon of rising *yang*. Here, extra attention is required to ensure that this

---

1   太極: The concept of the "ultimate supreme" in Daoism, or *yin* and *yang*, opposite polarities entwined with one another (symbolized by two stylized fish, most frequently in black and white). The martial art by the same name is based on this very concept.

2   陽氣 (*yang qi*): The *yang*, masculine aspect, from the balanced dichotomy of *yin* and *yang*.

3   一陽來復: The complete cultivation of *yang* energy in preparation for further practices.

yang is not intermixed with lustful energy or thoughts—only *yang* free of sexual thoughts is pure *yang*.

Under the guidance of an experienced practitioner, one can even go a step further, and begin to "gather medicine." Regardless of whether you are gathering the "small medicine" or the "big medicine"—both are foundational to Daoist cultivation and transformation of spirit and *qi*—the most important point is that at the outset, when you first enter meditation, you must take care to ensure that your mind becomes truly tranquil. This type of tranquility is not influenced by a state of stillness versus movement; constant vigilance is required either way. One must continually alert oneself and direct one's inner light of attention toward the mind itself. This is particularly critical when one is frightened or worried: take distance from the poles of good and evil, right and wrong, from every kind of differentiation. One must not let one's head be turned to dwell on past good or bad events. Return often to the mind, to listen and examine. In turn, put all that passes over the ears from the outside world between the coming and going of breath, and do not make false judgements.

When one has nothing to do, let the eyes rest half open and half closed, and focus them on a point. It does not matter what the external surroundings are; the only thing that matters is attention to regulating the mind and breath.

With regard to sleep, one should not force a certain length of slumber on oneself. It does not matter whether sleep is long or short; what matters is the depth of the sleep. Additionally, dreamless sleep is desirable, because through deep, dreamless sleep, *qi* can be cultivated and energy restored—kidney *qi* will be robust only if nourished with this type of sleep. Thus, before sleeping, remind yourself to put the mind to rest before closing your eyes. At this time, adjust the breath to facilitate relaxation. Relaxation must be complete, permeating throughout body and mind. You will then enter sleep as a matter of course. Focusing on the *dantian* area, you may even achieve unity of mind and breath, and the dreamless sleep of a sage. This then naturally gives rise to the cultivation stage in which the five *qi* types return to and nourish the mind, and the conception and governing channels are open and unobstructed.

Medical doctors have performed studies on primates to assess sleep quality. If the primates had problems adapting to the environment in which they were living, they would exhibit psychological distress, total insecurity. If the sleeping environment was not good, their sleep would be shallow, and they would remain partially vigilant while sleeping. Because of the lifestyle of most modern people, their sleep is also easily hindered, the main hindrances mostly owing to anxiety about life. People do not feel stable or secure; they are physically busy, their minds chaotic. Some people end up developing the habit of going to bed late as a result of efforts to relax their minds and bodies from their bustling states. They might stay up late doing things on the computer or watching movies, while others also spend time thinking about the vexing matters of their day-to-day lives. Harboring such bedtime habits inevitably leads to poor sleep quality. The solution is quite simple: find a method to return your mind to pure stillness. Always come back to stillness: enter tranquility, do not hold on to any thoughts. Release all illusions and judgements from your mental space, and single-mindedly focus on regulating your breath. Persevere in this, patiently practicing inhalation and exhalation. The natural result will be the enjoyment of unbroken slumber until daylight, at which point you will awaken feeling pleasantly refreshed. In this way, the body and mind will continually improve.

In the Daoist art of cultivating tranquility, innumerable are the mystical methods in addition to the previously described "Sixteen Gold Ingots." Among these, the most important is foundational attention to the three sacred treasures of the body: above all, focus on refining essence, cultivating *qi*, and nourishing spirit. It is necessary to know the central rationale that all past masters of Daoist internal cultivation understood. At a minimum, do not casually let your vital energies seep out. Cautiously guard your reservoir of life-force. To maintain fullness of essence, you must understand how to "gather the medicine" and draw upon the universe for boosts. Everything else has to do with how to refine essence and turn it into *qi*, how to refine *qi* and turn it into spirit, and, finally, how to merge spirit with the void. A new practitioner of Daoism and meditation must grasp the essential points about building and guarding full vitality in their own body. Otherwise, any teachings they receive farther down their path will be meaningless. Modern people are overly concerned with rapid progression; their essence has already been leaked in their teens, so many people are like this. Therefore, with meditation, the art of cultivation, and all of the basic training, the earlier one begins, the better. Most of you present right now have broken and leaky bodies. In fact, the critical challenge facing most of you is how to enhance your being and make it whole. You should even aspire to renew your body so that it is like that of a newborn: this is foundational.

A great number of people come here to study. When asked why they want to study the Dao, many of them reply that they wish to open the conception and governing channels. This is delusional, an impossible way to approach these matters.

When I was living on the mountain, I waited upon a few Daoist elders. When they were choosing new monks, almost all of them would ask whether the candidate was still a virgin. Furthermore, they would ask whether he had ever ejaculated, and whether they had ever had wet dreams. They questioned the candidates in great detail. And why did they interrogate them like this? The purpose was to determine whether they were suitable for this path, and to assess their basic potential for spiritual cultivation. Essence is the most important and foundational element of an individual. If the essence is weak, the *qi* will be deficient and the spirit scattered. In that case, how could someone become a receptacle for the Dao? Therefore, the most basic and critical step when beginning a meditation practice is to first make the necessary adjustments to the three treasures: essence, *qi*, and spirit. You must first establish your guard over your essence to prevent it from leaking out or being exhausted. To this end, stay away from sensual stimulations; do not be occupied with anything but nourishing vast *qi*. The key to not letting your *qi* leak out is to avoid speaking; and the path to nourishing the spirit is through lack of desires and cravings: to be natural in all things.

Take, for example, the Daoist elders who dwelt in the mountains. They began seeking the Dao in their youth. Ultimately, they returned to heaven and became immortals, and leading up to this transformation they essentially did nothing but meditate. Thus, to protect essence, *qi*, and spirit, the best method is the tried-and-true practice: persevere in sitting meditation; try to sit until your mind and spirit have unified, and the same *qi* permeates your mind and breath. Ultimately, the *jing* will be able to return to your brain and nourish it. The forefathers constantly gave the reminder that those who seek the Dao must not be bothered with other affairs; the foundational matter of life is to collect and conserve essence, protect *qi*, and regather the spirit. Once, in Sichuan, I met a Daoist elder who had been greatly esteemed by Du Xinwu. No one knew this elder's true age. It's been said that in the Daoist school very few people ask about dates of birth, because age is considered an outside matter—Daoists don't discuss it. Legend has it that this Daoist elder didn't leave footprints, and some other stories hinted that he had the power to rescue people from death.

Once, a certain tycoon was passing through Chengdu, and his wife suddenly fainted in her tracks. Her family was at a total loss for what to do, what the proper way was to revive or help her. Fortunately, some of Du Xinwu's admirers were treating the Daoist elder to a meal at a nearby restaurant. As soon as the news of the incident reached the dining party, the elder went to the woman's aid, and spoke with great feeling: "Please don't be anxious; she'll be fine!" He moved his hands in a flash. With the "sword fingers" of martial arts, he applied pressure to three acupoints on the woman's body. Immediately, she let out one great yawning breath, and her consciousness returned. In no time she was quite well indeed, chatting and charming everyone present. The tycoon's family members could not but kneel and bow to the elder, and they begged to be taken on as converts. From that time forward, the tycoon's whole family observed practices of Daoist cultivation and devoted themselves to good deeds. It is said that after the husband and wife began seeking the Dao, they started sleeping in separate rooms; they did not have intercourse for many years, adhering to asceticism and cultivation arts, building up robust vitality, their faces radiating light.

This couple had sincere faith in and devotion to the "Celestial Worthy of the Original Beginning."[4] Thus, on the celestial being's birthday, they would go together to the Daoist shrine in the mountains to show their respect and worship. I chanced to meet them on one of these visits. With great curiosity, I asked: "What are the daily teachings of your master regarding how to reach enlightenment?"

The tycoon replied earnestly and openly: "Our family's master constantly tells us to single-mindedly pursue the Dao and nothing else. We began on this path in middle age, and our initial practice was focused on regaining the vitality we had let seep out over years prior. Furthermore, we learned that *yin* and *yang*[5] energy cannot dwell together—to attempt to cultivate them both would certainly cause disaster. It's important to meditate for six hours every day, and cultivation should be practiced through self-restraint and refinement of the mind. Long-time dedication to sitting meditation will naturally result in the protection of essence, the transformation of *qi*, and the storing of spirit. Among ancient and modern Daoist immortals alike, there have not been any who did not begin by attending to these principles. All corruption must be avoided." These are the things the tycoon said the Daoist priest taught and demonstrated on a daily basis.

The tycoon once told someone that the Daoist priest, daily, would use the martial arts of *taiji* and *xingyi*[6] to instruct his juniors.

---

4 元始天尊 (*yuan shi tian zun*): One of a triad of most commonly worshipped deities in the religious form of Daoism.

5 陰/陽: The two opposite, complementary polarities that keep the body (and all of nature/life in general) in a functioning balance, according to the theory of 太極 (male/female, hot/cold, light/dark, etc.).

6 形意: Or 形意拳 (*xingyiquan*), one of the three main (internal) martial arts of the Wudang style (武當拳), the other two being *taijiquan* (*taiji*) and *baguazhang* (*bagua*).

Once, when trying to put in check a young and inexperienced fellow, he used the technique of levitation, lifting a large dining room table in the great hall of the tycoon's home. He let the table hover in space, dumbfounding all the young men present, who then knelt and began bowing repeatedly. They realized that this Daoist priest was no ordinary person. Thereafter, they all dutifully followed his every word, not daring to add a word to anything he said.

CHAPTER 8

HANDLE AFFAIRS HARMONIOUSLY, UNHINDERED IN BOTH MOVEMENT AND STILLNESS

Sifu said: "All these tales tell us that, regardless of the *gongfu* level of a practitioner, the emphasis is on the centrality of essence, *qi*, and spirit. These three exhibit differences in their prenatal and postnatal forms: in their prenatal form, they are called original essence, original *qi*, and original spirit. 'Original' here emphasizes the nature of being inborn: they are the original three treasures before any of them have been degraded or lost. After an individual is born, separated from their mother's womb, they will experience a multitude of feelings in reaction to a multitude of stimuli, and all sorts of confusion in response to a multitude of uncertainties. Gradually, the desires that affect an individual after birth will result in damages to, and leakages of, the three treasures of vitality. If the seven orifices of the human body are not guarded appropriately, and the individual does not have a master to guide them in the regulation of these apertures, postnatal *qi* will also be consumed. On top of that, bad habits in managing the seven emotions and various desires will lead to excessive consumption of spirit, and the individual won't be able to store their spirit *qi*. This principle underscores that the starting point of Daoist practice is the nourishment of spirit and vitality. Of course, there are many methods for spiritual nourishment, but the most important one is to abandon all pensiveness. Over the course of human history, there has been no shortage of noble men and seekers of the Dao, but why have so many of them yet died prematurely? The reason is they were unable to pacify their spirits, unable to abandon fame, wealth, and power.

Consider Emperor Taizong of the Tang Dynasty (born Li Shimin, 598–649). Though he eventually ascended to the throne, the previous rulers had made a shambles of the civilization, and he had to confront all the consequences. On top of that, he was involved with the grisly Xuanwu Gate Incident.[1] He was also generally occupied with devising strategic operations and overseeing the law and social order of the country. Consequently, for a period of many years, Li Shimin had almost no rest, becoming increasingly hot-tempered and irascible. When he did sleep, he slept lightly, was easily disturbed, had many dreams, and often experienced night sweats. This went on for some time, provoking a serious conflict and disorder between his fire and water elements. Eventually, he had what modern people would call a nervous breakdown. Thereafter, it was only after taking an herbal decoction from a highly skilled doctor of the time, Sun Simiao, that Li Shimin was finally able to sleep peacefully. This good fortune was due to Li Shimin's great karma.

In that time of peace and prosperity, there were many people of exceptional talent. What's better, during his time as Emperor, Tang Taizong understood how to select and promote the best and most virtuous men. He treated the wise courteously and cultivated the scholarly. The fruitfulness of that dynasty was beyond that of any Chinese dynasty preceding it. Of the doctor, Sun Simiao, it is said that he was truly in the Dao, and that in addition to his profound understanding of the healing arts, he had penetrated the spiritual realm. The emperor trusted him because whenever any member of the emperor's family encountered a difficult situation or began suffering a complicated illness, Sun Simiao's intervention invariably brought remedy to the issue at hand. One particularly notable instance was the pregnancy of Empress Zhangsun.

---

1   A successful coup attempt on 2 July 626, during the Tang Dynasty, for the imperial seat in Chang'an.

She exhibited strange complications, and all of the imperial doctors were mystified. Every medical professional in the palace gave up, so Sun Simiao was called in. To everyone's amazement, all he had to do was prick one acupoint, and the Empress smoothly delivered a baby boy. Naturally, Emperor Taizong was overwhelmed with delight, and he offered Sun Simiao a handsome reward.

Now, Sun Simiao had no interest in a privileged life of fame and fortune. He preferred to drift like a cloud in all directions, helping the distressed and destitute wherever he roamed. Sun Simiao authored the *Beiji Qian Jin Yao Fang* (*Essential Formulas for Emergencies Worth a Thousand Pieces of Gold*), which has since been handed down through the generations. It is the most important text in the entire canon of Chinese medical literature. Sun Simiao also made an invaluable contribution to the methods of internal cultivation practiced in orthodox Chinese Confucianism. Since he passed on to his next life, there has been an unceasing stream of posthumous titles conferred upon him from the rulers of the Chinese civilization. His legacy is also strong among the common people: many are the temples devoted to this immortal, and to this day they are flourishing, overflowing with visitors and offerings.

In Li Shimin's era, respect for Daoism was paramount. It was said that Laoshang Taijun[2] himself interceded on Li Shimin's behalf and bestowed his protection through countless disasters. Before Li Shimin ascended to the throne, he had been to worship the famous Daoist priest Wang Yuanzhi of the Mao Shan Sect. This priest was highly respected both by the government and the public, having been the favorite pupil of Daoist immortal Tao Hongjing. Because Wang Yuanzhi had long been acquainted with Emperor Gaozu, it was only natural that he would have an affinity for Li Shimin. Wang also imparted teachings in the law and methods of magic arts to Li Shimin.

---

2   太上老君: One of the "Three Pure Ones," the highest Trinity of Gods in the Daoist pantheon, pure manifestations of the Dao itself. Laozi is said to be an emanation of this.

History then turned to the Song Dynasty, in which many self-indulgent and fatuous rulers emerged. In that era, numerous Daoists hid on the sacred mountains of lore, sealing themselves off from the world. Only after a period of great struggle did fate eventually offer another emperor of any benevolence, Emperor Xiaozong, who understood the theory and practice of governance. He also enjoyed casual study of the sages' works.

In history, he was the most gracious of emperors, and went to incredible lengths to defend and uphold the decrees he believed would bring happiness to the people. He extended pardon to Yue Fei for the unjust ways in which history had treated the disgraced general. Simultaneously, he was harsh in his punishment of unjust officials. But among his attendants, Xiaozong did not have the good karma to come across an adviser of Li Shimin's caliber. The latter was exceptional in his fortunate encounters with a most capable individual willing to assist him in governance and even to forgo his seclusive way of life. Song Xiaozong, on the other hand, ultimately became entangled in solving economic problems, and for an entire decade suffered from serious insomnia.

Over the course of history, there have been many sovereigns who have not understood the principle of maintaining order through restraint, causing themselves disturbances of the mind and body. No shortage of them have been on tenterhooks, without peace. In fact, it doesn't matter whether speaking of kings or common folk, it is simply human nature to tend toward vain thoughts and rigid judgements if one has not yet begun on the path of cultivation.

If bad lifestyle habits continue over a long period of time, then the mind will churn chaotically and one's intention will be uncontrollable. This also results in excessive loss of essence, *qi*, and spirit. All those just beginning on the Daoist path should be taught to start by quieting their desires, which will clarify their natural disposition. Gradually, on the path, they will be able to extricate themselves from the vulgar conventions of this world and return to authenticity. They must not engage in any impure behavior;

their actions should take after those of a maiden, undefiled by the ways of the world, not giving people cause to raise their eyebrows at them. Remain calm even in the midst of vexation, understand when to remove yourself from circumstances of carousing, or any context that provokes bodily lust."

Sifu then spoke candidly about his own experience in the early stage of his studies, and he shared the origins of several teachings and certain exemplary cases from Daoist history. Through these explanations, he demonstrated the importance of essence, *qi*, and spirit in the study of Daoist cultivation and meditation. He also emphasized that the main point of meditation was not what one might think based on mainstream traditions of meditation, so many of which only amounted to blindly sitting in boredom. Rather, one must master the rationale underlying these exercises and grasp their true meanings, applying the principles in all areas of life. Whether busy or at rest, and in whatever posture, one must be agile and comprehensive in one's practice and advancement on this path.

From the moment we disciples came under *sifu's* guidance, he began stressing the point that meditation is just a process—we should not rely on it too much. The truly critical question is how you carry the practice of cultivation into your life after a period of meditation, and how you keep your physical body in the most excellent condition possible. Accordingly, *sifu* often remarked that the apex of Daoist cultivation was manifest in daily activity, that is to say, in successfully maintaining perfect tranquility throughout the regular movements of life.

Sifu told us that once as a young man in Sichuan, he had a chance encounter with a follower of Luo Chunpu's lineage of practice. It came up in their conversation that in his later years, Master Luo also stressed that Daoist cultivation was something that must permeate a practitioner's whole life. If you experience a transcendent connection with the Dao, you should not just isolate this realization in meditation and the sensory organs and bodily apertures. Instead, the realization must be made manifest in the form of *qi*, with which you infuse your every interaction with other people. Furthermore, every facet of your mind must be limpid and clear like a radiant moon. Your mouth must not speak of the rightness or wrongness of human affairs. Your ears will be deaf to sound and your eyes blind to the images of things. Everything that touches your tongue will taste like wax, and your body is forgotten since it naturally melds with everything it touches. Furthermore, you must understand how to meld your physical body with a relaxed mind, how to meld your mind with *qi*, how to meld *qi* with spirit, how to meld spirit with Heaven and Earth, transforming into nothingness.

Sifu told us that the conversation illuminated many things for him regarding how to cultivate the Dao without hindrance in both activity and stillness. He relayed these matters to the good-fortuned guests at the banquet table with great enthusiasm. Among them, Elder Lin seemed to particularly enjoy all that was being said, nodding along and sighing in agreement as *sifu* spoke. The main takeaway that evening was that although *sifu* stood by the importance of meditation, he put even more weight on what comes after meditation: the continuous practice of *gongfu* and preservation of vitality.

CHAPTER 9

A Patriarch of the Dragon Gate Sect Meets the Emperor

The School of Complete Reality has a unique history of continuous flourishing. True credit for this honorable achievement is due to one of its patriarchs and lineage holders, Master Wang Changyue. From my first encounter with the lineages of Daoism, I repeatedly heard Wang Changyue mentioned by the masters of my school, as well as other Daoist elders I visited. And at any such mention, there was no one among them who did not immediately bow deeply with folded hands, expressing their sincere esteem and respect. Why is it that today's Daoist disciples so venerate Wang Changyue? He is a legendary figure, a man of extraordinary wealth, who lived in the late Ming and early Qing Dynasty period and was a famous Daoist teacher. The wisdom he imparted belongs to the School of Complete Reality, his legacy intimately bound to the period in which he lived. He was born as the Ming Dynasty was coming to an end. Emperor Chongzhen desperately wanted to turn the tide, shake up the imperial courts, and pull out all the stops for a final fight. Day and night he attended to imperial affairs, and he did not avoid offending influential officials or root out bad actors among the eunuch faction in his efforts to save the dynasty. Although he was strict in self-discipline, he often revealed his vulnerable position in front of high-ranking officials. It is a pity that this leader of cautious mind did not come to the throne at a time of power, but rather as the final emperor at the end of a dynasty. His lack of a definite personal view and his tendency to hesitate before acting were the most important factors in the loss of Ming Dynasty rule.

Moreover, farmers all across the empire were hit with an intense famine—they did not even have rice to eat. All over the kingdom, people were engaged in bitter struggles just to seize wild weeds on mountain tops for sustenance. In their efforts to gather these weeds and mitigate their hunger, peasants ventured into far-flung, secluded areas. Some resorted to stripping trees of bark and boiling it in water in a desperate attempt to fill their stomachs. Yet more pitiable were those who had no option but to find some clean mud and eat it without anything mixed in. Because of these terrible circumstances, many peasants took advantage of the political turmoil to stage a revolt. The call to arms was raised from all corners of the land.

The period of crop failure and successive years of drought were followed by further destruction from a locust infestation. Truly, Emperor Chongzhen had a miserable fate as a ruler. During his reign of a little more than a decade, there was not one night where he could enjoy deep, carefree sleep, or a peaceful meal. The kingdom faced distress at home and invaders from abroad. In the end, the emperor could not endure under the pressure: with no other way out, he hung himself on Jingshan Mountain.

Wang Changyue grew up during this unstable period. He was immersed in evidence of impermanence and grievous events, and while still just a child, an extraordinary conception and pursuit of the Dao took root in his spirit. The moment he heard of any accomplished Daoist master dwelling among the sacred mountains, he would set off in the direction of that mountain top to visit the practitioner. In this way, he voyaged long and far across Northeast China. He visited dozens of Daoist masters, and eventually became the disciple of a Daoist priest from the Dragon Gate Sect of the School of Complete Reality, Zhao Fuyang. Zhao Fuyang was not one to accept disciples lightly, but Wang Changyue was humble and persistent, entreating him repeatedly. Zhao Fuyang saw that Wang Changyue's predisposition to Daoist cultivation was strong, and that he was close to divinity. Knowing that Wang was extraordinary, he accepted him as a student.

At the outset of this relationship, he earnestly said to Wang: "Pursuit of the Dao is not a simple path, but it is also not so full of hardship as one might think. From the moment you commit to this way, the most important thing is to use experiences of hardship and poverty to become a master. Devote yourself to all types of labor on behalf of others; serve the people. And I want to emphasize religious discipline most of all. You must devote yourself to perfect discipline, always following the precepts in your deeds and carrying out religious rites dutifully. Any free time you must dedicate to the important teachings I have shared with you, like those in the *Dao De Jing* and the *Zhuangzi*."[1] After Wang Changyue's venerable master shared this guidance with him, the disciple wholeheartedly concentrated on studying all of the scriptures and classical texts of Daoism, Buddhism, and Confucianism. This moment of instruction also set in motion the inheritance he would share with later generations of students through teaching and writing. During the next ten years of his life, he became even more serious about seeking out great masters; he roamed extensively through mountains and valleys to find them. Before long, his drifting took him to Huashan. There, he experienced a deep feeling of affinity and destiny of place, and thus went into seclusion on the mountain, shutting himself off from the world. During that period of isolation, he observed Daoist fasting practices and devoted himself fully to internal cultivation. He made great advances on the path, and drew near to the Dao. As a result of his discipline, he repeatedly experienced extraordinary correspondence.

Under his master's influence, Wang Changyue strove to revive the ancient School of Complete Reality's ancestral court. In compliance with the instructions of Wang Chongyang, founder of the School of Complete Reality, Wang Changyue re-emphasized study through monastic discipline. When he was teaching as a master, he presided over the ceremony of monk initiation many times,

---

1   道德經, 莊子: Two of the fundamental texts to both religious and philosophical Daoism, from the 6th and 3rd century BCE, respectively, authored by the legendary sages Laozi and Zhuangzi.

guiding over 1,000 disciples along this path. At the Baiyun Temple in Beijing, he converted numerous Daoist priests to the Dragon Gate Sect; not only that, but he himself voyaged out to the four corners of the kingdom to spread the unique teachings of the sect, and dispatched disciples to do the same. They took the wisdom of the Dragon Gate to Nanjing, Shanghai, Hangzhou, and many famous mountains. Slowly, under Wang's powerful and benevolent leadership, the legacy of Qiu Changchun, founder of the Dragon Gate Sect, came into a new period of flourishing, to the point that the sovereign at that time, Emperor Kangxi, began to revere Wang Changyue, and conferred upon him an official imperial title.

Nearly every follower of the School of Complete Reality has heard the legend of Wang Changyue's fated encounter with Emperor Kangxi. Every detail of this event has been vigorously debated and analyzed. It came about thus: Wang Changyue was presiding over Baiyun Temple, as ordered. During this time, he was observing strict ascetic practices, and had completely purified his body. All that he did was for the purpose of advancing on the path of the Dao. He entreated the ancients for their wisdom three times a day. Immortal Lu Dongbin was moved by Wang Changyue's devotion, and so, one day, he appeared to Wang Changyue in a dream and revealed a prophecy to him: "The emperor of the present dynasty, Emperor Kangxi, is going to disguise his status by dressing in plain clothes and venture out for a royal tour of inspection, and he will come, thus garbed, to Baiyun Temple. This is a fated opportunity for you to convert him; do not let it slip past you." Sure enough, the next morning, Emperor Kangxi quietly showed up at Baiyun Temple dressed in simple clothing and with no ceremony or announcement. None of the other Daoists in the temple realized that the emperor had come into their presence, but the sharp-eyed Wang Changyue recognized him the moment he saw him: the middle-aged man of uncommonly lofty bearing was indeed none other than Emperor Kangxi. Wang Changyue clearly remembered what Immortal Lu had conveyed to him in his dream.

To recount their meeting with more specificity, just as Emperor

Kangxi strolled casually into the temple, no one was there to receive him as a guest, but by happy coincidence, Wang Changyue was just emerging from the abbot's quarters and encountered him. Wang Changyue instantly knew in his heart the identity of the person standing before him, but he sedulously concealed his knowledge. He bowed politely to the emperor and greeted him. Wang was wearing a long robe of white, and his beard tumbled unrestrainedly down his chest. At first glance, Emperor Kangxi knew this was a man of great integrity and wisdom, a priest who was truly of the Dao. A feeling of great respect welled up in the emperor, along with a desire to question the priest about his beliefs. Kangxi proceeded to request that Wang Changyue draw hexagrams on his behalf, and the Daoist master obliged, going through the motions of hexagram-based divination. Wang Changyue then took up his brush and wrote a few words of interpretation, and presented them to Kangxi. When the emperor opened the message, he saw that this was no trivial matter—the Daoist priest was unusually resourceful, perhaps magical. A new motive emerged in Kangxi's mind. He could not let Wang Changyue continue to dwell in low stature so far from the imperial court. Thus, he put on a mild manner and continued to discuss Daoism with Wang, expressing his hope that the priest would offer him further guidance. In Wang's dream, Immortal Lu had provided lucid instruction regarding this exchange. In particular, Lu had told him he must not forget to address the matters of water and fire. Accordingly, Wang Changyue replied to Kangxi: "I thank the Emperor for gracing me with his favor. I am but a cultivator of the Dao, and thus ought not to have any material attachments. Today, his Majesty has asked if I have any requests. I have just one hope to mention—that his Majesty will grant me water and fire, these two things." When Kangxi heard this, he laughed inwardly, and thought, what difficulty is there to this? And so he agreed to Wang Changyue's request.

Following this encounter, tremendous turmoil came upon the capital city, owing to the hidden workings of the Eight Great Immortals: in just a few days, the water sources of every household in Beijing, including the imperial palace, dried up completely, and no kindling would light for fire. When night fell, all the people of the kingdom, be they royal or peasant, were left staggering about in darkness. Emperor Kangxi was a wise man, and the necessary course of action occurred to him naturally. He knew that Wang Changyue must be a reincarnated immortal and could not be taken lightly, so he made haste to dispatch an emissary to Baiyun Temple. However, it is said that once the aforementioned meeting with Kangxi had ended, Wang Changyue immediately left Baiyun Temple to return to Huashan. Thus, though the emissary sought the Daoist priest, he did not find him. But if one is searching among one's own rivers and mountains, who can be truly out of reach? Kangxi discreetly went out himself in his imperial carriage looking for Wang Changyue, thereby fulfilling the latter's wish to formally initiate people into Daoist priesthood. In later years, Kangxi personally oversaw the completion of this mission, and he granted more land to Baiyun Temple. Finally, Kangxi was initiated into monkhood under Wang Changyue's direction. This rare and marvelous sequence of events has since become legend in Daoist circles. The ancient master Wang Changyue wrote many excellent works, the most important among them *The Mind Skills of the Dragon Gate Sect*.

CHAPTER 10

TO CULTIVATE THE DAO, FOCUS ON ACCUMULATING GOOD DEEDS

On a certain weekend evening in the summer of 1980, I was at *sifu*'s residence. Despite the sweltering heat of that summer, the banyan tree at the entrance of the central courtyard was reaching toward the sky, and a low wall was covered in white osmanthus blossoms, flourishing. As I stood in the courtyard, a light summer wind, as if out of good will, whisked all around, filling the whole space with a sweet smell. He who dwelt here was so refined, a paragon of virtue, learned and advanced in the Dao—perhaps that's why the wind carried this fine fragrance of righteousness throughout the residence! In a word, every time I returned to *sifu*'s abode, in my heart I felt a sort of release from worldly pollution, as if I was transported beyond mundane matters. Although my body was still in the middle of a bustling city, it was as if I had entered another universe. The house was a Japanese-styled Western building of several hundred square meters. On ordinary days when *sifu* would lecture on the Dao, his room was like the abbot's quarters of Vimalakirti. Numerous people came and went from the house, bringing with them a crisscrossing of sentiments and attachments. The foot traffic of visitors was unceasing, like a steady flow of water, and yet there never seemed to be any obstruction in the space.

According to the usual schedule, Saturday evenings began with meditation. Thereafter, a senior student would lead some movement practices. Then *sifu* would instruct us. On the particular evening in question, however, *sifu* had Daoist friends visiting, so his usual presentation during the evening practice was canceled.

Eventually, some of the students dispersed. The only ones left in the residence were myself and a few other advanced practitioners who had stayed to help *sifu* receive the guests, and to generally offer assistance. Three elders from the Daoist circle came to call that evening. These men, all close, long-time friends of *sifu*, were from mainland China and had made the trip to Taiwan together. Among them was a thin, tall fellow of 70 years or so wearing a reform-era Chinese tunic suit. Two thin stripes of mustache embellished his upper lip, and his skin was swarthy. His presence was intimidating, a catalyst of awe and fear. However, observing him at the banquet, over tea and talk, my impression of him changed. As it happened, this elder, surnamed Ma, had a sense of humor totally unlike his stern outer appearance. This humor was especially pronounced in his retelling of anecdotes about Daoist immortals from ancient times. His hilarious accounts had everyone doubled over in laughter. That evening passed quickly, but even such a light-hearted occasion offered many profound lessons.

Elder Ma had been introduced to Daoism by the elderly scholar Fang Wuchu. On the evening when we were gathered at *sifu*'s residence, Elder Ma candidly described some of his fated experiences with Daoism. He too was a priest, and had entered discipleship under one of the official heirs of Min Yide of the Dragon Gate Sect. Min Yide is a central figure to the Dragon Gate Sect, having first encountered the Dao through a Daoist of the Jizu branch who converted him. This master was one of the heirs to Wang Changyue's wisdom—thus, Min Yide can also be considered to be part of Wang Changyue's Daoist lineage. This Daoist elder Min Yide was proficient in Confucianism, Buddhism, and Daoism. He was well versed in the histories, scriptures, philosophies and other classical works of all three. Furthermore, he had a profound and advanced practice of internal cultivation. His book *Transmission of the Heart-Lamp from Mount Jingai* is a master work of the Dragon

Gate Sect, and is considered the most detailed text to come from the school in modern times. In my own reference material, much is derived from the written works of Min Yide. His contribution to the Dragon Gate Sect of the School of Complete Reality is of true eminence. He put painstaking care into the writing of *A Compiled Daoist Canon*, which has been continually passed down since. This work has been of outstanding benefit to subsequent practitioners of Daoist breath regulation and cultivation of *qi*. With regard to classical texts on internal alchemy and cultivation and reference material on oral tips and other matters, his works are exhaustive. In his *Collection of Ancient Books from the Tower of the Bookish Hermit* alone are countless pearls of wisdom and rare teachings.

Elder Ma recounted: "I became a Daoist early in my life. I was once employed as an orderly in Hubei by a family who worshipped the God of Northern Heaven. Because of their faith, they made a pilgrimage to Wudang Mountain, and I went with them. I knew that Wudang Mountain was a holy place for the God of Northern Heaven, and I was full of enthusiasm on the pilgrimage, climbing the mountain with great zeal to pay my respects. Who could have predicted that on that journey I would meet my future teacher, a direct inheritor of Min Yide's wisdom! Of course, he was a monk in the Dragon Gate Sect of the School of Complete Reality, but he had come to Wudang Mountain because he felt an affinity with the place. He liked the natural surroundings and the spontaneous, non-action[1] Daoist energy of the mountain. When I encountered him, he had taken lodging in one of the mountain temples for the night. I was exceedingly pleased to learn from him about the Dragon Gate Sect of the School of Complete Reality and the teachings of Wang Changyue. I was especially compelled by the idea that one could enter a greater realm of reality and simultaneously renounce the world, and that these experiences could be melded together.

---

1   無為 (*wuwei*): Laozi explains that beings (or phenomena) that are wholly in harmony with the Dao behave in a completely natural, uncontrived way. This is the goal of spiritual practice, according to Laozi: the attainment of this purely natural way of behaving; effortless and spontaneous movement.

The teachings and rationale on proper comportment in society also attracted me. It seemed that the teachings of Wang Changyue could be applied to anything one might encounter in life, and that their significance only deepened with experience. Master Wang had said: 'From childhood, people study the so-called Confucian principles: propriety, righteousness, honesty, shame, etc. Why is it, then, that only a few people among the multitudes truly embody these virtues? If it is so rare and difficult to become a good person, is it even possible to become an immortal, to merge with the Dao?' These words took deep root in my heart and strengthened my affinity for the Dragon Gate Sect. The master I met on Wudang Mountain could see plainly my intensely favorable reaction to what I was learning about the Dragon Gate Sect. One day, he helped me compose a letter of introduction, and instructed me to go to Guan County in Sichuan province to call upon his friend Li Jie. Only later did I realize that this was Daoist Elder Li."

Elder Ma sipped tea as he recounted his unexpected connection with the great master Li Jie: "This great master Li Jie was highly proficient in the literary arts, and he was not only a scholar but also a gentleman of great virtue. In my opinion, in the past 100 years, he is one of the purest treasures to have emerged from within the schools of Daoism. Many people are unaware that he was a distinguished scholar, not to mention highly advanced in the *gongfu* of Chinese shadow boxing. When he was growing up in his village, he encountered a talented practitioner who instructed him; through the *gongfu* of his legs, this teacher could tread upon snow without leaving a mark. Great master Li was devoted to his people and nurtured a profound sense of justice. Early on, during the Manchu takeover, he was critical of the rulers' decadence and sluggish leadership. He was one of the first patriots in the Alliance Society [founded by Sun Yat-sen] to gain respect. He did mighty things in Sichuan, and whenever his name reached the Qing court, they trembled in fear. Later, for various reasons, the great master was moved to renounce the world, and so he summited Qingcheng Mountain. This man had a sunny, affable disposition and a grand aura about him. His most special characteristic was his hearty laugh, which one could hear preceding his physical arrival by many miles. The people on the mountain top adored him, and his own Daoist master gave him a new monastic name: The Joyous Priest.

Elder Li rarely spoke of his past, but everyone in Sichuan knew that he had passed through miserable, unlucky experiences, and that he had been through the travails of broken family life before eventually taking up internal cultivation and entering the Daoist order. After becoming a Daoist, he extricated himself completely from these external bonds and desires, and he refused involvement in any of the trivial affairs of the itinerant wanderers. Over just a few years of dwelling in the mountain forests, he was able to make a thorough investigation into the Daoist alchemical and *gongfu* practices for immortality and other areas of Daoist medical science. Because he had been steeped in *gongfu* practice since childhood, his later investigation into the Daoist arts and his strict ascetic discipline were magnified in effect, and the level of his powers soared. He accumulated a wealth of skill and strength, and he knew that he could serve all of society and even save lives with this *gongfu* and the fruits of his cultivation practice. He descended from his mountain top dwelling, and thus began his fated period of roaming the sacred mountains.

Elder Li's healing *gongfu* practice was distinctive. The power of his pinky finger was especially famous. When he encountered an especially difficult case, perhaps involving mixed and complicated symptoms, he would concentrate all of his internal *qi* into his pinky, and transmit healing through that little finger to the patient. The efficacy of this technique was extraordinary. The nail of this pinky finger he kept quite long, and sometimes it even curled up. There are a few accounts of this finger being instrumental in his treatment of stroke patients. He would use it as if it were an acupuncture needle, locating the relevant acupoints on the body of the stroke sufferer and pressing deeply. The results were miraculous. After hardly a moment of this healing *gongfu*, the patient would be able to get up and walk. Once, there was a villager who was crossing the road while carrying a heavy load on a shoulder pole, and a small freight truck hit him. He was all but crushed, and his foot in particular was shattered. Due to the limitations of medical treatment at that time and in that area, his wounds were tantamount to a fatal disease. But Elder Li treated him using *qigong* and all the traditional medical skills he had studied, applying several medicated plasters, and eventually the man was able to walk again just as before.

Elder Li was also highly learned in the astrological arts and fortune telling. He did not even require someone's surname to correctly divine their fate. Using only the 'Four Pillars of Destiny'—that is, an individual's birth year, month, day, and hour—he could interpret that person's palm. He became famous for this prowess in divination to such an extent that even important officials and celebrities heard about it, and all of those who did immediately sought his advice for themselves too.

Living in the same era, the renowned warrior Du Xinwu was among the lofty personalities who endorsed Elder Li. Du Xinwu was an eccentric celebrity in his own right. His attainment in *gongfu* can only be described as supernatural. During Sun Yat-sen's involvement in the Alliance Society, Du Xinwu served as his personal bodyguard, and it was only by Du's protection that Sun was able to avoid several attempted assassinations and other potentially fatal calamities. Song Jiaoren, however, was not so fortunate. Du Xinwu, Tan Citong, and several other stalwart revolutionaries had a strong bond of friendship, so when Tan Citong was beheaded by Empress Dowager Cixi, Du Xinwu was determined to avenge his death. However, Du's attempt to assassinate Empress Cixi failed, so he went into exile, roaming far and wide. Many revolutionaries and secret societies held him in high regard at that time, from the Heaven and Earth Society to the Green Gang. It has been said that even the big shots from the Green Gang considered him an authority. His prestige was evident everywhere. Even big-shot Du Yuesheng of the Shanghai coastal territory was considered his junior.

Although Elder Li had no contact with fringe vigilantes, his reputation preceded him, and all sorts of folk heroes admired this mysterious and towering character of the Daoist community. I was extremely fortunate that under the guidance of the elders in my family I was able to study with such a teacher. As mentioned, Elder Li was a master of divination, so all of his disciples were required to study and understand the *Yi Jing*. Additionally, to follow Elder Li's teachings on asceticism, internal cultivation, and the path to immortality, students had to have intensively studied the logic of the hexagrams of the ancient Daoist practitioners. Otherwise, it would be impossible for them to engage with the *Cantong Qi*[2] or other important classics. In his guidance of my studies, Elder Li also demanded that I rigorously and continually apply myself to The Four Books: *The Great Learning, The Doctrine of the Mean, The Analects*, and *Mengzi*, as well as other texts from antiquity. And every morning, I was required to rise between 4.30 and 5.00 am, to prepare for the morning meditation that took place from 5.00 to 7.00 am.

Under Elder Li's guidance, I learned a great deal about meditation and the Daoist arts, including the midnight–noon ebb–flow cycle, and how to transport *qi* within the body. However, after several decades of practice, I realized that there were a few things even more important to focus on than meditation or the macrocosmic or microcosmic orbits; that is, building up skill and virtue, and advancing in the cultivation of the temperament. Let me give an example: in Elder Li's teachings, we were often reminded that one must begin from a position of deference and humility. It is essential not to cling to a high opinion of oneself, and no matter the context, whatever time or place, one must never become complacent, but rather always seek areas for self-improvement. In one's conduct, one must never be hasty or restless, nor cause others anxiety, and one must not chase after sensual pleasures. Simplicity and stability must be the priorities of one's life. To cultivate the Dao and engage

---

2 參同契: One of the classics of Chinese literature, dealing with Daoist alchemy (內丹, *neidan*), from the 2nd century CE.

in scholarly inquiry, one cannot simply pick and choose, improving one aspect of oneself but neglecting others. In matters of karma, one must vigilantly guard against a sense of fear or dread; following the natural course of action in all things, one will not swerve from the course.

Finally, one must commit to lifelong cultivation of benevolence, justice, etiquette, and wisdom. If a person has a meek and loving heart, this shows a tendency toward benevolence. If someone has a strong concept of shame, and of good and evil, this is the principle of justice at work. If a person is not anxious about their own success or benefit, but rather has a habit of putting others ahead of themselves in all things, this is a demonstration of proper etiquette. As for wisdom, it can be found in the person for whom the distinctions between truth and fiction, uprightness and evil, are as clear as the reflection of a mirror.

Elder Li often admonished students of the Dao that in day-to-day life, one should nourish a sympathetic and careful way of thinking, and in this way increase one's chances for good thoughts and good actions.

After I came to Taiwan, my fate was such that I met people from all walks of life—scholars, peasants, business people, all sorts—and from encounters with such disparate people, I experienced a great range of personalities and dispositions, and was willing to find mutual encouragement with the virtuous. I learned to not strive for wealth among those who hoard material treasures; to not seek prestige among the rich and famous; to not vie for fame among the pretentious; to not argue with the haughty and rude; to not contend with the arrogant.

The Daoist elders I met among the mountains as a young man told me that those on the path of Daoist cultivation should not dwell on superfluous concerns involving right and wrong, love and hate. This is the direction practitioners take in order to make discerning judgements."

CHAPTER 11

ON CESSATION OF THOUGHT FOR A QUIET MIND, AND THE CORE THEORIES OF VITALITY

Elder Ma had certainly attained the Dao—he spoke with a strong, clear, and resounding voice and was in high spirits. Listening to him talk transported me to a Sichuan province teahouse, decades in the past. Among the few fellows that had stayed back that evening there was one classmate, Li Shande, a Chinese doctor who lived on Zhulin Road. Because he lived not far from *sifu*'s home, he would regularly take it upon himself to serve him. He was quite an erudite scholar himself, in his sixties. Still diligent in his studies, indefatigable and never slacking on the path of the Dao, he elicited the favor of *sifu*. And he took advantage of this rare opportunity to ask Elder Ma some questions he had concerning this path of practice.

"This humble student has been practicing meditation under the host master's guidance for several years, but still struggles with one issue, though I regret to bother the teacher with such a question. However, an audience with the magnanimous, honorable teacher is truly difficult to come by. Therefore, I boldly ask whether I may request his advice."

Elder Ma modestly sought *sifu*'s gaze, and my teacher graciously signaled his approval with a wave of the hand. Li Shande proceeded: "I am quite ashamed; even though I have practiced Chinese Medicine for many years, I personally have continuously struggled with nocturnal emissions. I understand this is related to excess fire and deficiency in the water element of the kidneys,[1] and have even effectively prescribed jade lock pellets[2] for this imbalance in my patients. But although this treatment works for others, it hasn't worked for me. It seems like I alone cannot overcome this issue. I have been wanting to ask for *sifu*'s advice on this issue for some time, but I felt inhibited. I thought, this is such a small issue, I should not dare to bother *sifu* with a trifle."

Elder Ma replied: "This is actually a common concern. In my younger days, I also worried terribly about this issue, and I came to suspect that my struggle with it may have a karmic root. After settling on that theory, I didn't bother focusing on the matter. However, in my peripatetic period, I had a lucky encounter with an old traveling Daoist monk who showed me a method that I think is quite useful. Since then, I have had absolutely no anxieties over this matter. The method he taught me is simple: every evening before sleeping, cross your arms on your chest; then, with all the strength you can muster, inhale and bring your *qi* into your *dantian*; as you inhale, forcefully contract your anus, as if in an urgent attempt to prevent defecation. Practice this a few times, and it will have the desired effect. There is one other method that can be practiced each time you need to pee: lift your heels, and urinate in controlled, separate spurts; open your eyes wide, do as if you were fuming with rage: raise your head with eyes wide open, and clench your teeth."

Sifu sat to one side listening as Elder Ma detailed these practices for self-regulation. When the latter had finished, *sifu* described one more method: "When you are going to bed, take care not to shut all the windows in your bedroom too tightly. A few windows should be left open enough that fresh air can flow in. Before you sleep, sit up straight on the edge of the bed. Rest your hands naturally and gently on your knees, and bring the tip of your tongue to your palate, behind the top teeth. Thus positioned, practice breath

---

1   相火過旺，腎水不足 (*xiang huo guo wang, shen shui bu zu*): In Chinese Medicine, this refers to reduced metabolism and endocrine function caused by poor nutrition, errant fluid control, and excessive heat of the body.

2   玉鎖丹 (*yusuodan*): A type of Chinese medicine prescribed to resolve the problem of nocturnal emissions.

regulation. When you have reached a relaxed state, forcefully inhale fresh air through your nose, and direct the inhalation to your *dantian*. Then, from your *dantian* area, slowly bring the breath back up and expel it through both nostrils. This must be practiced many times, but it is very helpful for dealing with the difficulty you mentioned."

After *sifu* had finished describing these techniques, he was concerned that some of the students present might not be able to understand the method, so he got up from the banquet table and took a seat on a tatami mat to the side. Sitting there, he delved deeper into his explanations, using hand gestures to clarify the method. After this demonstration, he returned to the table. He then addressed the student who had asked the original question, offering some final points of clarity on what he truly needed to progress in his earnest practice:

"Although the meditation practices all seem identical for all, they will actually bring into play the good deeds and merits of each practitioner's past life. The process relates to the depth or shallowness of this well of blessings and virtue. Some people are able to open up the flow of *qi* in their bodies after just ten days of practice. In your case, I have explained clearly to you many times what your biggest challenge is. You should focus on accumulating good works, serve others without seeking reward, and think less about these bedroom concerns. Worrying about the latter will hinder your opportunities to connect with the Dao. Your spiritual constitution is inherently deficient. If, moving forward, you do not use the cultivation practices to address these deficiencies, you will pass through this life in vain.

Hearing you ask your question today revealed to me that you are still stuck at a certain stage of cultivation. You need to learn how to refine your essence and turn it into *qi*, and how to transport that *qi* throughout your body. Right now, there remains a blockage in the movement of your *qi*, that is, in the area below your *dantian*. At this point, what you need most is to incorporate the principle of 'pure intention.' To begin with, as I have mentioned to you before, it is of utmost importance in meditation to start with cessation of thought. If your mind is churning, the practice is futile. Although you are rigorous in your self-restraint, these maladies still arise. The kindling that lights this overwhelming fire will cause you much grief and will be of no profit. This state is what people are talking about when they say someone strays in this practice. The fact that you have been practicing meditation for many years but still habitually leak semen shows that you have not let go of your thoughts about sex. This is the seat of your malady; you must consider this root to address the problem and benefit from the practices. At present, the only thing to do is return to the starting point. Apply your utmost effort to mitigating thought and quieting the mind until 'inside nothingness, pure, prenatal *qi* is suddenly apparent.' Before you enter that state, you will have to find a way to dissolve your desires, otherwise you will continue to fall short of the ultimate goal.

The majority of the problems modern people face in trying to progress in their meditation practice is that they carry too much heat in their lower abdomen. Whenever *yang* rises, they can't suppress it. I've often seen all the gains someone has gleaned from a month of meditation dissolve in an instant because of this, and they may hit this block repeatedly, so that even in their old age they have not been able to progress and achieve greater success in the Daoist arts. Special attention is required for those who begin on the path of meditation practice. If the practitioner's *dantian* area exudes a heat that extends to the four limbs or the whole body, if the two kidneys are extremely warm, at this time the perineum and lower abdomen will be very comfortable, and particularly if the testicles are taut. If the practitioner experiences any of these sensations, then critical attention is required, and he cannot slacken in willpower for even a moment, otherwise leakage is sure to occur."

Although *sifu*'s tone during this speech was somewhat stern, it was clear that he was making these statements with a sincere and benevolent motive: to share the truth and offer earnest advice to Brother Li. *Sifu* often rebuked us young and inexperienced disciples, but always with good intentions. He never gave up on us, reminding us tirelessly of the most important principles to abide by in meditation. In this instance, *sifu* even went so far, in his great kindness, as to demonstrate how to strengthen the kidneys, the fundamental theories of vitality, and preservation of the *dan*[3] through avoidance of leakages. To this end, he taught us the "Garuda Spreading Its Wings" practice, as follows:

"The two feet must be shoulder-width apart, and the whole body relaxed. When beginning the exercise, breathe slowly. A certain amount of warm *qi* will gradually ascend from your *yongquan* point up to between your kidneys. Then, when you inhale, raise your heels, and do as if grabbing the ground with your toes—use your intention to clench the toes, do not use force. Simultaneously, raise your arms to the sides, as if spreading your wings open to fly. This exercise was passed on to me by a Daoist priest I encountered during my time in the mountains. He shared with me that it was only after he had already married and settled into family life that he began practicing Daoism. Consequently, early in his study of meditation, he still often ejaculated unintentionally in his sleep. Around that time, he encountered a monk from Wutai Mountain who taught him this exercise, and also mentioned that another useful practice is to tie knots on a white rope while reciting mantras to bless it, then tying it to one's waist while sleeping. This mitigates leakage even further. The monk said that he had done this for many years, and it had proven effective."

---

3   丹: The immortal pill produced through Daoist inner alchemy, a very high level of practice which, when successful, ensures a long healthy life and entrance into "immortality"—not so much an endless earthly life, rather an ultimate merging with the immortal Dao, with all that is.

CHAPTER 12

AN INTRODUCTION TO THE INNER ALCHEMY PRACTICE OF QUIETING THE MIND

A smile began to appear on one half of elder Ma's face, listening to *sifu* as he began and nodding his head in agreement. Having listened to *sifu*'s instructions and enthusiastically brought up his experiences of the core techniques he once studied, he then conveyed these same methods to those of us present.

"I learned this practice from a disciple of Master Luo[1] I met in Sichuan, who told me I could employ it if I were to experience leaking of essence when meditating. As all the movements of this practice are done standing, it is considered a type of posting. For all of you in attendance, if you feel disturbed in any way during seated meditation, there is no harm in using this method to adjust your mind, and to assist your practice in areas that are lacking.

It is extremely simple. Standing, place your feet shoulder-width apart. Using your intention, starting at the top of your head, lead all of your body's dirty *qi* straight down and let it exit at the *yongquan* points; your knees should be slightly bent, but they shouldn't extend past your toes. Breathe in and out a total of three to seven times. When you breathe in, all your toes should very lightly grip the floor; when you breathe out, relax and allow your toes to return to their original position. Continue by rubbing your palms together until hot, then massaging your kidneys 36 times. Your palms need to be on the lower back, over the kidney area, and your intention should be focused there, as well. Return your mind

---

1 Master Luo Chunpu, referenced in Chapter 8.

to the ebb and flow of your breath, until the mind and your breath become interdependent and uninterrupted.

When you breathe in, use your intention to bring your *qi* from the *yongquan* point up along the governing channel running up the back of the body: starting at the sacrum, up past the *mingmen* (in the middle of lower back, opposite the lower *dantian*), through the *jizhong* (lower back, top of the lumbar spine), then the *dazhui* (upper back, top of the thoracic spine), the *yuzhen* (back of the head) acupoints, and up to the *baihui* (at the crown of the head), then down to the *renzhong* (just above the teeth). When you breathe out, follow the conception channel running down the front of the body downward, passing through the *tanzhong* at the center of the chest and the *zhongwan* just below solar plexus, then stopping upon reaching the *qihai*, just below the lower *dantian*. Note that when practicing this method, there is no need to go all the way down to the *huiyin* at the perineum. Finally, gradually bring your *qi* all the way down to the *yongquan* point. This is done in one breath cycle. With the next inhalation, do it again, moving from the *yongquan* up the back and down the front. Repeat this cycle three to seven times. Use your intention to move and guide your *qi*. When doing this, you must pay attention to a few things: the inhalation should be relatively longer while the exhalation should be relatively shorter. When you stop breathing, hold it firmly at the *dantian*.

If you do this over a long period of time, you will certainly attain the ability to concentrate the mind until it is single-pointed and supple—*yang qi* will then naturally develop. If you have a knowledgeable teacher to guide you, when the moment to pluck the medicine is before you, you will notice it. Keep in mind that when you practice, you must do so until you are completely focused and away from affliction, desire, and temporal distractions, until the mind and body are empty and thoroughly relaxed. Only then will your efforts yield fruit."

Afterwards, *sifu* also called attention to a principle to apply while sitting: when regulating your breath, you must breathe slowly, finely, deeply, and without interruption to the best of your ability, but you must be methodically balanced. When you breathe in, you must visualize that the five elements[2] of the universe transform into the five colors. These colors are like a rainbow, gradually entering through the nostrils. After entering into your body, take the five color fibers, connect them with the body's essence, *qi*, and spirit, then move them down into the *dantian*. After a while, you will certainly restore your *yang qi* and sexual potency, and create vitality. During this process, those who are sensitive may experience soreness or numbness during practice. These sensations can be ignored. After practicing this over time, the micro- and macrocosmic orbits will naturally open, and the eight extraordinary meridians and twelve ordinary channels will naturally be without blockages.

And one more thing I should mention: after *sifu* finished explaining these tips, the attention shifted to a man we knew as Senior Chen, a man in his seventies who had accompanied Elder Ma to the gathering. Senior Chen contributed his experience: he had been practicing the "12-Step Brocade"[3] every morning upon waking, combining it with other techniques from the *Yi Jin Jing*[4] transmitted on Wudang Mountain. He spoke emphatically of a Daoist classmate of his who had practiced his whole life in this manner. Already 102 years old, he still had good ears and eyes, and could read and clearly distinguish the characters of a newspaper even when the font was extremely small. He didn't need presbyopic glasses, and his limbs were nimble without impediment, just like a young man's. Upon asking him how he was able to attain such a healthy state, he had replied it was due to the very practices that Senior Chen spoke of. This evening was indeed an extraordinary

---

2   五大元素 (*wu da yuan su*): Earth, water, fire, air, space.

3   十二長生功 (*shier changsheng gong*): Also known as "12-Step *Qi* Bathing Techniques for Longevity," a set of "*qi* bathing" exercises, illustrated in the Practice Guide and Exercises in Part 2.

4   易筋經 (*yijinjing*): A Daoist *qigong* method that can be translated as the "Tendon Transformation Classic."

and happy occasion for all those who attended—we all received precious practices and instructions.

For many, the process of Daoist practice of "refining the pure" entails searching high and low, painstakingly, all for the sake of finding the perfect formula that will bring about the golden elixir. Because of this, they will not hesitate to spend their every penny traveling far and wide in search of a wise teacher. There are also quite a few who become urban hermits, or build a straw house and live in the mountains, just to attain accomplishment and return to their original soul, their original nature. However, they are helpless, their reasoning unclear; wise teachers are difficult to come across. Most individuals will go to a bookstore and pick up two or three books on the subject that are written by modern authors, and after returning home, they will copy what they read—in the end, many of these people will also be led astray. In the practice of the Dao, the difficulty lies in cutting off one's desires. Nearly eight or nine out of ten people are not able to stick to this principle. In order to suppress their desires, some people will use incorrect methods. In the end, the vacuous fire of the five viscera and six bowels will flare up and, thus, the result is self-defeating.[5] All the great, virtuous masters of ancient times, and those who had mastered the arts of longevity, never lived in violation of the principles of *yin* and *yang* and the laws of astrology, divination, and face reading. Their lives were altogether ordinary: they never overexerted themselves physically, never left the body malnourished, and followed the ways of nature to cultivate the wondrous qualities of spirit. This is quite different from modern people's habits of enjoying a night-life of singing, eating without restraint, and drinking carelessly. They get dead drunk every night, having drunk sex, hurting their bodies, destabilizing their essence, using up their spirit, looking

---

5   五臟六腑之虛火旺盛 (*wuzang liufu zhi xuhuo wangsheng*): It is said that vacuous fire occurs internally as a result of excessive sexual desire or an over-abundance of scattered thoughts. Thus, it's implied here that suppression of the desire is insufficient to transform the internal regulation of the elements and organs.

for happiness in the wrong places and living excessively in their everyday life. After 50, they will show significant signs of aging.

The concept of *xian*[6] in Chinese lore refers to those who achieved immortality through the transformation of their essence, *qi*, and spirit—that is, turning one's essence to *qi*, followed by accumulating *qi* to preserve the spirit. Once the spirit is full, longevity is achieved. The three stages have to be completed to perfection, which is not an easy task, to say the least. To build the foundation, practitioners ought to reach the preliminary step of the merging of *kan* (water) and *li* (fire). When cultivation of *yang qi* has progressed to its mature stage, it is called "jade liquid reversion elixir." I've witnessed many of my senior and fellow practitioners who went through a lot of trouble in order to advance the practice of the microcosmic orbit, only to fail because their concentration began to waver as they were confronted with their temperament and desires. The importance of meditation-induced erection in Daoist practice lies in its primordial *qi*, a practice called "returning to the *yang* from extreme *yin*" in the *Yi Jing*. When the stage of "returning to the original nature" is accomplished, one can enter the macrocosmic orbit, which is followed by "shifting the furnace and cauldron," thus successfully obtaining the pill.

My Daoist practice hasn't reached a point where I feel adequate to share my insights with others in order to be of benefit to them. But if I were to allow myself, I would say that—whether one devotes oneself to the practice of Chan Buddhism, Vajrayana Buddhism or Daoism—nothing can surpass mind training. This is according to the many years of experience gained by all my predecessors. For succeeding at training the mind, the foundational Daoist practices must be completed in full, otherwise something will still be lacking. According to Daoist traditions, transforming one's essence, *qi*, and spirit requires single-minded attentiveness, to the point that if any delusive thought or ego-clinging arises,

---

6   仙 (*xuan*): Commonly translated as "immortal," though it does not carry the same meaning of eternal life as in the West.

practitioners will have to go back to the beginning. In other words, for both experienced and novice meditators alike, initial progress is made with the death of the mind. Note that "death" here does not connote stagnation; instead, it refers to the state of a mind that is clear as a mirror, capable of penetrating insights yet giving rise to no differentiation. If one can reach such a state in one's meditation—combined with the building of the foundation through 100 days of abstinence, nine years of wall-facing focused retreat, and three years of supplementary cultivation—such a practitioner can attain a modest level of achievement.

There have been a few practitioners who fervently seek the three methods of the so-called *san yuan dan fa*.[7] Without wasting any time discussing whether the heavenly alchemical method is even still obtainable or not, it is a fact that those practitioners who were said to understand the other two methods have long passed on. On top of that, these alchemical practice methods simply cannot be replicated by modern theories of chemistry or physics. In ancient times, practitioners were said to be able to transform stones into gold, taking elixir to achieve immortality and resolving worldly problems for people. Currently, this is lore that can only be read about in books. Even if we were to delve into external, earthly alchemy—how to consume foods that are beneficial and appropriately nourish our physical body to avoid illnesses—we would inadvertently enter a rather muddled and confused territory, where opinions on the most basic methods of achievement vary greatly, and no unanimous conclusion can be drawn. Are we to even venture into the complexity of the other two alchemical methods, the "mortal" and the "heavenly"?

The ancient Zaijie and Qingjing Sects both had specific practices dedicated to Daoist alchemy. However, the terminology used is often cryptic, and one absolutely needs a qualified master who can explain it and properly induct the aspiring practitioner.

7　三元丹法: The "three fundamental alchemical methods" of Heaven, Earth, and mortals.

And even if one were to fully understand all the terminology, aren't we running the risk of encountering the pollution of modern substances and soil? Truth be told, the "heavenly alchemical method" can be divided into external and internal alchemy. Based on realistic assessment of the current conditions we live in, the safest practice method would have to begin with the inner alchemy centered on clarity and non-action.

CHAPTER 13

WHEN THE MIND IS UNHINDERED, ACTION AND STILLNESS ARE UNIFIED

The ancient Confucians described true self-possession: one who has realized this virtue does not complain when complaint is justified, does not react with anger when provoked, does not hold forth just because an opportunity to speak arises, does not rejoice when met with delights, and is not startled by any alarm. The individual who demonstrates this degree of restraint can be considered to have a peaceful mind. They have reached a suitable state from which to begin the practice of meditation. When entering meditation, if the sitter integrates the principles of letting go of afflictions and not being attached to external circumstances, adjusting the breath appropriately, then thoughts and insignificant matters will dissolve naturally into emptiness.

The term "sitting" in "sitting meditation" implies the melding of all regular hours of the day with those spent in meditative practice. That is, times of practice and non-practice are unified in true "sitting." When sitting encompasses every hour and every day, the subtle flame of *wen* [the mind's intention] can emerge, and the myriad things will be illuminated.

A person new to the practice of meditation should very cautiously approach the observation of their consciousness, as if they were handling their very lifeblood. I am referring here to the practitioner's relationship with their mind. Look first for answers in the silence of meditation. Gradually, as the cacophony of voices in your head diminishes, this state of cautious observation will clarify.

This is the road that steers straight between extremes, wherein lie divine conduct and sincerity of mind.

From a person who lacks this sincerity of mind, all is contrived. The most critical factor in internal cultivation is to hold oneself to seeking the truth. The "truth" that I am referencing is the true mind. When this true mind manifests everywhere, then the practitioner has become pure. Not a single speck of dust stains them in this state, and their mind cannot be hindered or led astray—this naturally leads to harmony of *qi*. A meditator must reach this realm of tranquility at the beginning of their journey, and within it, they should distance their mind from all illusions of terror and flights of fancy. After much persistence in practice, they will arrive at a place in their cultivation where they face no more obstacles or hardships.

To wholly let go of the mind is to bring forth the sincerity for realizing the true mind. When the mind has been released and abandoned, the recluse who dwells on the most remote forest peak loses all distinction between the walls of the temple, and the wilderness. When the mind has been released and abandoned, the practitioner who lives amongst the chaos of worldly trappings won't fall into reveries of prosperous olden days. No longings can overtake the person whose mind is truly set at rest. Even if they travel far, they will not daydream of home.

Adherence to this practice of quieting the mind through meditation will result in total clarity of being, with no trace of the false world left. Even the slightest illusions—those that usually cling like a fleck in the eye, or a tiny seed stuck in the teeth—will have no hold on the practitioner who persists in this way. On the throne of the spirit, not a sliver of impurity can remain.

When a Daoist practitioner is not seated in meditation and walks amongst the mundane world, their mind must not be disturbed by gain, loss, ruin, or acclaim. If any such thoughts enter the mind, the practitioner's pure tranquility will turn into base appetites, and they will slip far from holiness. The mind should be empty, free from all impurities. The consciousness can then encompass all of Heaven and Earth, as broad as the cosmos itself.

This is how a meditator should practice. Only then will their ease and confidence extend without limitations.

During meditation practice, concentrating the will with full attention is key, but it's important that the resultant tranquility not be confined to periods of sitting meditation. The practitioner must maintain absolute serenity off the cushion too, whether in movement or stillness, sitting or reclining. If the mind remains unmovable while the practitioner is active, this shows that the mind and breath have reached stable interdependence. That is to say, at this level, one can practice breath regulation during periods of regular activity.

Those who understand the microcosmic and macrocosmic orbits know that these circuits do not simply adjust themselves without discipline. For modern people, the negative effects of today's technology and the many pollutants and noises of the environment require extra consideration in this practice.

If neither "no mind" nor "quiet mind" are within your grasp, do the practice of "restoring the gentle lord." Indeed, if one who has not reached these states stubbornly persists in meditating, then the subtle and physical body will suffer all sorts of corruptions. In particular, vacuous heat will overtake the five viscera and the six bowels. If the practitioner is negligent, they may seriously enfeeble their body before ever manifesting the Dao.

I studied at *sifu*'s home for many years. Advanced Daoist priests regularly came and went from his residence, always discussing Neo-Daoist teachings on quintessence. However, it seemed that this focus was at odds with the real world. One may single-mindedly persist in breath regulation, *qi* circulation, internal alchemy, and *chao yuan* ("returning to the origin") exercises, amassing all sorts of theories and terms in the practice of *gongfu*. However, if the practitioner completely ignores the secular world and meditates blindly, then they will not understand their own pursuit. It is unwise to go through the motions in ignorance. Not only will the practitioner struggle to progress in the Dao, they will also be putting their life in danger.

Seekers of the Dao need to understand that implementation of these teachings should accord with practical circumstances: Daoist cultivation must evolve with the times. Changes in material culture and the greater environment should be accounted for in the modern practice of internal cultivation. People must act pragmatically within the context of their era, otherwise they will not be able to support interconnection among the six roots. This approach is also necessary to prevent intention and spontaneity from impeding each other, and to maintain the discipline of "forgetfulness" between states of action and stillness.

There was a particular Daoist elder who had been a general in the army. He spoke about the countless posts he had held over the course of his military days, and how fortune had saved him from calamity. Even under heavy fire, he often emerged unscathed. In his younger years, an old Daoist in his hometown had taught him to count his breath and meditate. He became extremely adept at these practices and eventually used his skill to heal himself of two gunshot wounds, as well as an older affliction of the bones. Truly, he reaped much from his meditation practice.

He often said that the greatest blessing of his life was having the chance to study the wonders of meditation from a knowledgeable teacher. In almost every free moment, adhering tightly to the oral tips, he would adjust his breath and settle into meditation. These frequent sittings had almost become his normal state. He meditated through the night rather than laying down to sleep. He said he kept no superfluous objects in his home. His room only had one narrow mattress, which he sat upon during his evening meditations. His diligence in self-cultivation was evident.

He once spoke of the many maladies he suffered before he began practicing meditation. He traveled far and wide, seeking out famous physicians to help cure him of the sores and wounds that covered his body. He tried acupuncture, herbal decoctions, ointments, and various other treatments from both Chinese and Western Medicine. But after each treatment, the slightest change in the weather would send him spiraling back into pain and distress.

He wasn't comfortable resting in bed, and he couldn't walk properly. At his worst, he couldn't even muster the strength to hold up a bowl.

Later, he began studying meditation, and after three months, many of his ailments had cleared up. When the weather changed, most of his previous pains no longer bothered him. After he had been meditating for half a year, all of his suffering had lessened. Most miraculously, after a full year of practicing meditation, his backaches completely disappeared. His legs, which had troubled him to the point of rendering him immobile, became strong, and he could walk for miles every day without the slightest effort. Even his farsightedness was cured. Because of these experiences, he became enthralled by the techniques of Daoist internal cultivation. He pursued his interest zealously, using any free time during transfers between military posts to seek audiences with master teachers. During these visits, he received a wealth of precious oral tips.

This was all well and good, but the fellow's circumstances changed for the worse after he arrived in Taiwan and retired from the military. His misfortunes began when he met a certain divorced woman. Thereafter, he drifted further and further from the way of Daoist cultivation, not to mention the lessons of meditation that he had been studying so earnestly for the better part of his life. He withered and became sickly. All of his old ailments returned.

Only later did he learn of the aforementioned woman's unusual history. To support herself, she had entered the world of brothels and dance halls. She later married a playboy she met during her career as a dance girl. The retired general was not aware of the many blights on this woman's character. She was an inveterate gambler, and through this habit she had squandered all her savings from her work in the dance halls. Her husband disappeared, and old age caught up to her. In these later years, her only option was to work at a friend's restaurant.

One day, the old general invited several of his former military comrades to dinner, hosting them at the restaurant where this woman was employed. The general was an old friend of the

restaurant's owner, and through this connection and the pleasant-
ries of that evening, the working woman and the general got to
know each other. Their interactions became more frequent, and
eventually they became an item. In and of itself, this is no matter
for criticism, but the dark side of the situation is clear from the big-
ger picture. This man had lived most of his years as a soldier, nearly
always busy with military affairs. Before he was born, his parents
had made a preliminary marriage arrangement for him, but he had
no experience in pursuing partnership or affection on his own.
Consequently, he found women difficult to understand.

By contrast, the woman had been shaped by her background:
she had become accustomed to living as a prostitute, with a different partner in her embrace each night. This former dance girl had
quite a way with men in general, so a fellow like the old veteran,
nearing his twilight years, was all too easy for her to manipulate.
Because the man lacked worldly experience, he did not consider
that first impressions might be misleading. He hadn't taken in the
old adage that time and experience are the only clear lenses by
which to see people's character.

The general didn't bother to look into the woman's past at all.
Knowing nothing of her previous relations, he followed his sensual
impulses and quickly gave himself over to his new feelings. In less
than half a year, they had registered as a married couple. He had
no idea that within a few months, the woman's previous lovers
and ex-husband(s) would come looking for her at their home
and harass them. The general was dumbstruck by the constant
stream of unwelcome visitors, not knowing how they had gotten
information on his wife's whereabouts. In addition to this troubling
development, the 30-year gap in age between the general and his
wife became a source of difficulty. He began to feel frustrated in
every aspect of their relationship—their differences in culture,
background, and personality all grated on him.

The woman was glamorous and had an attractive figure. She
had always gotten a lot of attention in the dance halls, with no
shortage of doting patrons. No wonder she wouldn't want to give

the time of day to the old general's charmless ways and plain talk. As a result, she went out frequently, sometimes spending nights elsewhere. Her behavior vexed the old man, who felt powerless. He was at a total loss as to how to properly address the situation.

It all played out as one would expect. The woman had begun avoiding her new husband early on, and eventually she totally disappeared. The general couldn't get any word from her. In his years of Daoist cultivation, he never touched cigarettes or alcohol, but the pain of this brutal blow drove him to almost daily drunkenness. He also slept poorly. At first he used alcohol to numb himself, then he developed dependences on various drugs, self-medicating to get through each day and night.

I was shocked when I last saw him. This was not the distinguished southern gentleman I had met before. Gone was the lofty air of the general who had led thousands of soldiers to glory, gone his expansive pride and boldness. I had met him several times before this all came to pass, and he had always left a favorable impression. Seeing him again later on, I was dumbstruck at his grim transformation into a tottering, shabby old man. His desolate countenance bore no resemblance to the spirit I had once seen in him. It was terribly pitiful.

CHAPTER 14

HOLD ONTO THE PRECEPTS, RETURN TO THE SOURCE— TRANSFORM THE PHYSICAL AND THE SPIRITUAL

After all of this, I heard *sifu* and a few Daoist practitioners who had come to Taiwan from Shanghai bring up a similar story again over casual conversation. One of them had been a businessman in Shanghai, an older gentleman who later put aside his career to pursue the Daoist path. He recounted the story of a wealthy woman from Shanghai named Lin Daiyu. She had been christened by the local media at the time as the most famous prostitute in the city, having used her feminine graces to cheat an immeasurable amount of wealth out of her male clients. Countless were the victims of the spells under her skirt, from religious figures, to working men of various trades and walks of life, to celebrities and merchants. Reportedly, even a provincial commissioner, in a moment of magnanimous abandon, gifted her a garden villa, despite only having known her a short time. But despite the lure of this crowning achievement, Lin Daiyu had no intention of leaving her trade for marriage. To the contrary, she spent half of her lifetime dangling this same carrot of matrimony to lure other men into scams, a game in which she was successful nearly 20 times. Eventually, she vanished without a trace, along with the money.

The details of her legendary life might leave one speechless and astonished at how deeply greed can root itself in a person's life and actions. One time, with her eyes on a large sum of gold, she was even willing to become someone's mistress to obtain it, but ended up having a dalliance with that person's servant instead. Lin Daiyu pulled her wiles all from the same bag of tricks. First, she ensnared her target's heart with the allure of beauty. Once she had him in her grasp, all of the jewels and gifts lavished onto her would be turned into cash before she locked it away into her own accounts. She kept her assets…diversified by spreading them all over Shanghai. Scams were not her only suit; she would sprinkle the stolen cash amongst her gigolos to keep them full, happy, and entertained.

It was such that she spent her golden years living on borrowed luxury. Later in life it is said she became desolate. With the constant stream of unscreened "guests," it was not long before her body, beset by venereal disease, underwent great change. With the passing of years, her sex appeal faded as quickly as her looks. In middle age, she was indeed already an old woman, with one foot in the grave. She later died miserably of illness in a dilapidated old apartment, alone and unattended.

In regard to this collection of stories, a few of the Daoist adepts brought up the importance of a practitioner's temperament, especially when guarding oneself against sexual desire, and conducting oneself in private life. In the undertaking of "complete chastity and sleeping alone," if you wish to practice the way of purity but are unable to keep a firm hold on inner and outer phenomena, you would need to apply the keeping of the precept of consciousness and guarding one's "trueness," a principle great practitioners of the past remind us of.

> *A young pretty maiden might be frail,*
> *Yet she can kill a foolish man as if a sharp sword hung by her*
> *waist;*
> *The man's head might not be severed from his neck,*
> *Yet his vital energy would all be consumed*
> *Till only a bag of bones remained*

Although this is a cautionary poem, it is indeed true to life.

From ancient times to the present, preserving, replenishing, and protecting against leakage of essence has been the primary aim of Daoist training, in accordance with Daoist formulations: as long as you can contain your essence, it becomes easier with time. If, however, you exhaust the spirit, and expend the essence, at best case, you shorten your life span; at worst, you bar yourself from accomplishing the Way. If you aren't able to preserve your essence into middle age, then what use would meditation be to you, even if you were relentless in your practice? The method of preservation is just as it is stated in the ancient texts: "Avoid exhausting your spirit and essence."

I often hear the words of such and such a person who has given tips about supplementing what is lost. Whilst each school claims its particular methods for preventing leakage of essence, in truth the correct way had already been dictated long ago by the immortals of the past, known as "collecting primordial essence," that is, collecting the inner *qi* and returning to the lower *dantian*. Other methods that are superficial fixes to the mistake unequivocally present some dangers. On top of this misinformation, consider the rarity in modern times of qualified practitioners who truly understand this path, and it becomes even more paramount to emphasize that, under no circumstances, in the race to the glorious summit, should you ever neglect the well-trodden trail. The real way of nourishing essence into *qi* should entail following a regular diet, keeping yourself collected and restrained, and cutting down on desires; nothing to do with chasing after shadows and mysteries in your room. This is the real peril!

As stated in the *Mengzi*,[1] "If it receives its proper nourishment, there is nothing that will not grow." Furthermore, it is said that the highest level to which you can practice retaining essence is to be blind through seeing eyes, deaf through hearing ears, to remain untouched and unspoilt as a virgin. Free of disturbance from what is external, and with the mind always quiet and abiding in stillness,

---

1 孟子: Also known in the West as *Mencius*, one of the foremost books on Confucian philosophy. Authored by the eponymous Chinese philosopher and sage from the 4th century BCE, considered second only to Confucius in the pantheon of Chinese thought and philosophy, and the latter's *de facto* successor.

it is only a matter of time before the cultivation of essence and *qi* will be within your able grasp.

The few great Daoist practitioners with whom I studied actually managed to preserve their physical purity up until their passing, a feat which is nothing short of incredible. Over the course of 10 years following and observing my *sifu*, I never once witnessed a moment when his gaze fixated on any female student or visitor. He would always keep his eyes locked on a point on the floor in front of him, never taking a sideways glance. All through the mirth and flow of conversation he would remain this way, unmoved. He never allowed himself to be alone with a woman in the same room, and had never once in his life even held a woman's hand.

I remember a time *sifu* asked: "The fully shrunken genitalia described in Buddhism: have you seen this before?"

I answered: "Of course not!"

Many years later, as *sifu* was nearing the end of his days, he called me over to his side. He said: "This time, and this time alone. There will not be a next." Inhaling, he drew his genitalia in until they looked like an infant's; exhaling, they returned to normal. I stood there, wide-eyed and speechless, thinking I had just witnessed some kind of magic.

Every Daoist practitioner must take their own path, but the hardest among them is "pure practice"—living a simple life, while cultivating one's character and progressing in one's spiritual practice. There is no need to discuss "attaining immortality"; among the committed individuals I have met in my life on the Way, rare are those who could even be called pure, and of few desires!

Once, when I first met a certain handsome Daoist adept, a man from Zhejiang named Ren, in his features I could instantly discern the air of an achieved practitioner. His face was refined and chiseled like polished jade, and his youthful complexion glistened with spiritual brilliance. I learned that, at one time, he himself had built a retreat hut in the Yandang Mountains, near his hometown, to practice stillness.

The Yandang Mountains stand out from China's southeastern

mountain ranges as peaks of historical prominence. They have been a beacon of homage for many of China's literary greats, and were appraised in Xu Xiake's *Travel Diaries* as the only place fit for practitioners of Daoist immortality. The range has indeed become somewhat legendary, with so many mystical and wondrous stories springing from its hidden landscapes over the ages—for a long time it has been a fortification for the propagation of both Buddhism and Daoism. Anyone who alights there on any regular day would be instantly transfixed by the smoky greens and hard reds wrapped in dark mists, speckled with bright blooms. It is just such a land that bears the holy traces and marks left by Buddhist and Daoist masters who found ultimate achievement within it.

It is the same otherworldly quality of those peaks that inspired our practitioner Ren to undertake focused retreats there whenever he had any time for himself. His footsteps were heard on such sacred spots as Hezhang Summit and Guanyin Cave. He was particularly fond of meditating on rocks just beyond the torrents of waterfalls, maintaining how tremendously beneficial it was for his practice. His only complaint was not being able to experience such bliss at all 18 of the range's sacred places of practice. One thing he did not regret was, in his early years, happening upon one of the mountain's Daoist sanctuaries, a place steeped in the powerful spiritual energy of its surroundings. It was there that he met the master who would transmit him the pith instructions and oral tips of Daoism.

Daoist brother Ren seemed to be in high spirits during our exchange. Perhaps we had a karmic connection, but whatever the cause, he opened up with his personal experience of practicing *yang* and cultivating *yin* in his lower abdomen, giving a careful explanation of the *qu gui liu ren*[2] method for male potency. With great care, Ren shared his knowledge while at all times keeping his words in accord with the Daoist doctrine. He said: "This is one of the secret teachings of the Way of Immortals, one that you do

---

2   去癸留壬: Literally "removing water/yin while retaining qi/yang."

not need given your young age. Nonetheless, since you seem to have a connection with this practice, I have decided to follow the circumstances that have unfolded, and give you a general account of this method. It is one that middle-aged men would most likely find useful. Attempts made by those in their more undisciplined youth could result in regular leakage, a habit that could lead to graver illness."

The method explained by Mr. Ren takes one to two months of daily, focused practice. It involves alternating use of the intention and gaze to guide the governing channel. Though he explained this in great detail and I jotted down absolutely everything, I actually never encountered any of the complications. The years slipped past, and now a few yellowed pages of old notes is all that is left.

As I grew older, through the perusing of Daoist literature I inevitably encountered techniques from the Southern School on how to replenish one's essence. Perhaps partially due to my personality, or the influence of my Daoist master, I never spared too much attention to study such techniques, preferring instead the mode of practice advocated by the Qingjing Sect of the School of Complete Reality. There are, in fact, myriads of practice methods—the key essentially lies in whether practitioners can achieve the perfect emptiness and stillness, along with their capacity to examine and reflect.

All books on Daoist alchemy detail *yang qi* as arising only upon reaching an extreme state of stillness. Only the true *yang qi* that is produced from ultimate emptiness and stillness is qualified to be called such, and by token, only the primordial essence produced thereafter can be considered true essence. This is precisely the point patriarch Lu Chunyang once made about transforming one's *qi* by utilizing primordial *yang*[3] in order to ascend from a mundane to a supramundane form. This is the state only Daoist practitioners with a high level of attainment can comprehend. An ordinary person will have no way to understand why primordial

---

3   元陽 (*yuanyang*): The portion of *yang qi* that was already present at birth.

yang can only be produced under the highest state of emptiness within emptiness.

In more modern terms, this means that once a person has become sexually active, and begins to think about and desire sex, their essence becomes impure. In other words, it can neither be refined nor extracted for later stages of alchemical practice. It is only possible to generate primordial essence before such desires and thoughts arise. If an experienced teacher is available as a guide who can prevent the student from getting carried away by desires, said student will have the potential to practice purely. Their essence can be transformed into original *qi*, which, if able to ascend, can result in the attainment of the state where essence and *qi* do not leak from the body.

One's meditation practice should begin from the gradual building and holding of single-minded focus, unifying one's essence, *qi*, and spirit. It needs to become a habit, and can be built by its liberal application to all daily activity until one attains a mental state of complete and utter stillness in which the spirit congeals, the *qi* gathers, and essence rises. This cannot be achieved without collecting and observing one's mind throughout the day, or during seated meditation. You can start by training the mind to become motionless. Begin by observing the ins and outs of the breath until it gradually becomes long, subtle, soft, and continuous. When it becomes effortless, and the mind and body have become settled, relaxed, and stable, then this is the miraculous result: the mind is motionless, the spirit does not wander, and the essence does not escape.

One should not trouble oneself with all the obscure Daoist techniques and formulas such as "requesting the secret of the tenth Heavenly Stem" or the "exchange of Heaven and Earth," what is the "real lead" or how to "utilize the cauldron." For the past few decades, many have been the requests to explain these matters. To all of them, I have given my universal reply: "There is nothing that can be said." Why so? Because there's really no need to take a risk out of desperation to seek methods that are outside of your mind.

For people of this day and age, it is quite sufficient, and without any potential risk, to simply focus their efforts on meditation and observing the breath.

Whether it's sitting or moving meditation, your first checkpoint is achieving the state of non-differentiation between the ego and the other, and merging with the world. At this point, the practitioner's *yang qi* will naturally develop, signaling a need to increase the amount of time spent in sitting meditation. Meditate until an erection occurs, then rub the hands together until they're hot. Place one on the kidneys and one on the navel, all the while gently placing awareness on the kidneys. Some of the instructions from centuries past stipulate that this exercise is best performed between the *zi* time period (11 pm to 1 am), though there are those who say it is not tied to a certain timing. It really depends on one's physical constitution, and the thoughts that come when one's *yang qi* rises. There's no need to be attached to it; simply regulate your breath until it becomes as solid and immovable as a mountain. Only then will the miraculous nature of the School of Complete Reality show itself.

The greatest secret of the School of Complete Reality lies in the pure, uncontrived mind, free of cravings. Only when the spirit is full can perfect emptiness be attained—ultimate focus without disturbances is key. This is the real meaning in the phrase "roaring dragon among rising clouds and the vermillion bird closing its wings." To achieve the ultimate goal of Daoist alchemy, one must first be able to unify the body and mind, complete the total transformation of one's physical and spiritual being, until eventually the physical and spiritual forms are no other than one and the same. Only when these three aspects are present, can one's Daoist alchemical practices bear fruit.

CHAPTER 15

MEDITATION SECRETS TO STOP EXTERNAL DISTRACTIONS

I remember two days before *sifu*'s 70th birthday, I received a call from my elder disciple Shenglong: "*Sifu* has been hit by a car. Many students are gathered at his residence. Can you come quickly?" I was hit by a wave of anxiety, thinking of *sifu* being elderly and where he had been injured. Was it serious? Thus, taking long strides I quickly jumped into a taxi, and headed to *sifu*'s place in Yonghe.

When I arrived at the estate, I saw a dense crowd of old students. Some had furrowed brows, others bore an expression of deep concern. Some were busy helping deliver water, some were preparing items according to the master's instructions. Stepping through the entryway and onto a tatami mat, I saw *sifu* reclining against his mat. I immediately put my hands together and bowed respectfully to him, then listened to the senior disciple's account of the event. Even though he was badly hurt, *sifu* maintained his characteristic demeanor of warmth and kindness, and acknowledged me with a nod of his head. I soon learned that, earlier that day, *sifu* had gone out to make a prescription for a sick person. While he was on a crosswalk, just before reaching the other side of the street, a taxi swerved to avoid hitting a pigeon and struck *sifu*, sending him to the ground. Most senior citizens involved in such a sudden car accident would have found it intolerable, let alone had their pelvis been fractured and dislocated as it was later discovered was the case for *sifu*. This type of injury is usually sent to the emergency room and would render most people unconscious or even kill them. However, not only did *sifu* refuse to make a fuss, he didn't even demand compensation from the driver or start an argument with him. Enduring the pain, he slowly walked back to his residence. It was only later that a female student on duty noticed that *sifu* was moving slowly and with an unusual gait. She became concerned, but *sifu* made little of it and casually said: "I was crossing the road and was accidentally hit by a car. The bones are possibly broken and dislocated. But don't fret or worry! Go notify some of the senior students at the medical clinic to come give me a hand." An elderly person's fall is a very different thing from a young person's. Indeed, their calcium levels quickly drop, which creates serious osteoporosis. It is very important for them to avoid traumatic injury and falls, otherwise they are susceptible to many hazards such as comminuted fractures. They may require an operation, and even if they are able to recover, they may still have ensuing complications as a result.

Many experienced doctors have said that the aftermath of a hip injury is a very serious, and in some cases even a fatal, condition. This is because of the long time it takes to heal and the immobility it incurs. Many people during this time develop bed sores or urinary tract infections. There may also be complications in the veins of the lower body. If not treated carefully, it is a great threat to life.

This event that happened to *sifu* gave me an even deeper respect and admiration for him. Afterwards, I heard a senior disciple say that *sifu* relied entirely on his own strength and traditional skills to set his bones. He also made a plaster from an old secret recipe, as well as his own anti-inflammatory, analgesic, and bone-healing medicines, which allowed him to heal in an incredibly short period of time. Throughout the entire rehabilitation process, I never saw *sifu* show any sign of embarrassment. He stayed in good humor, received the same endless flow of visitors, and never once lost his composure. He wouldn't let his ailments trouble others, and except for a few days of being slightly hindered, acted as though the event had never occurred. This level of resolve and self-reliance are the sunflowers of the elders I have held in my heart with the sincerest gratitude throughout the course of my life. On observation, we see certain Daoists who have practiced over 50 years, with perhaps 20 or 30 years' meditation experience, yet their mind remains unsettled. They are quick to blow a fuse and this harms their physical health. One of *sifu*'s Daoist contemporaries, who had established temples in the community, authored many works, and had many followers, came from a famous family, and had many good relationships, but he lacked patience. He always found fault in others, and even though *sifu* had long advised him against this habit, he stuck to his ways and never changed. One day, he got angry with his disciples over some publishing issues that he blamed them for. That evening, during his meditation session, he suddenly fainted. He was sent to the hospital, but had left this world before he even reached there. *Sifu* would often use this example to remind us that the most important point of meditation practice lies in the quietude of our mind and temperament. Lacking this can be extremely dangerous, as it is easy to go astray and encounter grave difficulties. *Sifu* proffered a wealth of warnings and instructions, but as concerns the practice of stilling the mind, I believe the oral tip "restricting the outer and containing within the center" is the most crucial. During the state of meditation, as well as entering and exiting it, you must not dwell on the past or let your mind be disturbed by external things. The mind must be in a state of complete and clear awareness, otherwise it will become muddled and scattered. If you continue to practice in this deluded state, over time illness will develop. Therefore, *sifu* would frequently quote the classics and invariably discuss methods of abandoning the seven emotions and six desires, harmonizing *yin* and *yang*, settling passions of the heart, and developing clear contemplation, etc.

CHAPTER 16

INDIAN MEDITATION—A SPOKE ON THE SAME WHEEL

I myself have spent a considerable amount of time practicing meditation, learning under a range of schools and techniques. In addition to meditation from Vajrayana Buddhism, I also studied traditional Kundalini yoga from India and *tummo*,[1] exchanging techniques with many masters. During this time, I also saw and experienced first-hand many wondrous, inexplicable things, from the likes of people so fantastical they could have been characters of fiction. Take, for example, the late Daoist master Liu. A seasoned meditator and alchemist once paid him a visit at his temple, a scene which I witnessed personally. Having become so accustomed to sitting for almost three decades, this meditator reported feeling as though his governing and conception vessels were constantly blocked, unable to be opened. Master Liu, hearing this report, simply picked up a toothpick off the table, and told the old meditator to settle his breathing. He then gently inserted the toothpick into the acupuncture point around the tailbone. Inconceivably, this small prick instantly and completely opened up the meditator's vessels.

An Indian master, a holder of the direct yoga lineage of Patanjali, was once invited to lecture in Taiwan. According to the representative at his branch in Taiwan, this Indian master, as a young man, had spent almost the entirety of his time seated in meditation. He once had one of his close disciples bury him in the ground, where he remained for an entire week without recourse to a single

---

1 　拙火 (*zhuohuo*): A yogic practice in Tibetan Buddhism where a practitioner learns to raise his body temperature in order to burn out impurities and remain unaffected by environmental conditions while practicing in retreat.

breath. This master had indeed already reached a high aptitude in meditation.

It was my fortune, through an invitation from another individual of the same school, to have the occasion to meet with this master in the 1980s. The Patanjali lineage, which he held, indeed has its own set of precepts and rules for cultivation. Although they emphasized sitting meditation, they believe that in order to reach oneness through meditation, you must subject yourself to a set of internal and external precepts as well as the purification of your mind. Only in this way can you reach the utmost heights of yoga. Whether through *asanas* or *pranayama* practices, his system's main goal was unequivocally turned toward attaining the union of Heaven and Humanity, in order to attain transcendent wisdom. In fact, after numerous interactions with traditions outside of Daoism, I felt that the thought and methods advocated by the religious traditions of the world's various ancient civilizations differed in form only, and tended toward the same goal. By looking closely into Indian meditation methods and the Daoist methods of refining essence into *qi*, *qi* into spirit, and then returning spirit into emptiness, I came to the understanding that they were spokes on the same wheel.

Indeed, the ancient meditation methods and essential instructions of India are strikingly similar to the internal alchemy of the Complete Reality school of Daoism: namely, returning to the state of the True Individual (i.e., an "immortal"), and to the ultimate state where everything returns to its original nature. It's just that the Daoist system has been laid out systematically, and a great congregation of achievers, all of whom demonstrated their miraculous supernatural feats, crowd the annals of Chinese history. In my youth, I had the utmost admiration for the Daoist master Ge Xuan, who developed supernatural abilities after receiving secret instructions and training from Immortal Zuo Ci in essential Daoist scriptures such as the *Jin Ye* (*Golden Elixir*). He holds a position of high status in Daoism, and is revered as the founder of the Lingbao School.

I have heard an unusually large number of stories on the

miraculous deeds of Master Ge from the elder generation of Daoist masters. It is said that when he was in a good mood, he could enter into a deep meditative stillness and stop his breath for several months at a time. He could spout water out of the top of his head, and fire out of his feet. His students would report meeting him in different locations, all at the same time. Most likely this was the ability of physical manifestation Master Ge gained upon reaching the highest levels of Daoist practice. It is said that he had the ability to turn stone into gold. He would often pull out raw copper and place the pieces into a small bowl, shake the bowl around a few times, and instantly the bowl would be full of copper coins. He would then give the copper coins to people in need. He could also summon celestial beings from Heaven to descend to Earth, allowing normal folk to see them with their own eyes.

All religions share the ultimate goal of liberation, as opposed to their adherents merely attending to the needs and powers of their physical form (which will eventually become a corpse). Whether in Buddhism or Daoism, supernatural abilities are steps along the way, not the end goal. Be wary of neglecting the foundations in a race to the peak, only to find you have squandered your life on ghosts and tricks. Much as the phrase goes, "Though there are many avenues to enter, there is only one road that returns to the Source," so it is that Daoist meditation, alchemy, holding the essence, and refining the spirit are all conveniences leading to the Way. Something that all Daoist practitioners understand is that the search for truth begins with one's own mind. The highest form of alchemy is to create spirit from essence. If there is insufficient essence, *spirit* will not be abundant, and will be unable to transmute, not to mention return finally to *emptiness*. Therefore, the ancestors guided their followers to first take up the practice of tranquility and *wuwei* (non-action).

In everyday life, you must put down the swirl of your million thoughts, and dismiss both suffering and happiness. With no wants and no desires, only then can you begin adjusting the mind and breath, and take a step closer to eliminating the notion of mind and perceived phenomena, and "forgetting" the dualistic notion of subject and object. Frankly, this is a more advanced method of refining essence, building *qi*, and nourishing spirit. However, in any case, you must start by nourishing the spirit with "no mind." Only then will you be able to enter into the primordial state of Dao. Daoist adepts of the past often said that in the initial stages of meditation practice, one must practice sitting until not a single thought arises, or "not a single speck of dust settles." Gradually, conditions arise where one's essence can be transformed into original essence, *qi* can be transformed into original *qi*, and spirit finally becomes original spirit. It may sound clichéd, but actually all these skills arise in large part from the depths of sitting meditation. Within both the Confucian and Daoist schools, nourishing the *qi* and spirit begins from the quieting of desires. The main points consist of maintaining your health, preserving the essence and the *qi*, along with the practice of observing sexual abstinence to gradually restore lost *qi* and spirit to their fullest. Only then can such a practitioner enter the Way.

CHAPTER 17

THE "12-STEP BROCADE" TO MOVE *QI* THROUGHOUT THE BODY

Although *sifu* had run into this bout of illness, he made a miraculous, speedy recovery and before long was active again. On a weekend that happened to coincide with our community's monthly gathering, I rushed over to *sifu's* residence a little early, perhaps a quarter past seven, as was my habit. I happened to see *sifu* in the courtyard, vigorously doing some stretching exercises that I had never seen before. They appeared to be some kind of gymnastics for the elderly, but were done very slowly. After I respectfully bowed to *sifu* with my hands together in front of me, I quietly stood to one side, and waited for him to finish his routine.

Sifu said: "This exercise is very suitable for older people or those recovering from an illness, and is a very effective *daoyin*[1] set performed after meditation to help the whole body's channels flow smoothly. The original exercises came from the School of Complete Reality, but I later made a few alterations, considering primarily those people who lack a foundation in meditation or who are very busy. Just with this one set of exercises, you can spread your *qi* smoothly and evenly throughout the body, just as well as during meditation."

After hearing *sifu* explain it this way, I found myself feeling very excited and immediately faced *sifu* to plead in earnest as to whether I could call on his compassion to teach me. He replied: "I

---

1 導引: A precursor of *qigong*, and practiced by Daoists for health and spiritual cultivation. Also commonly refers to a set of *qigong* practices.

can, sure I can. But you will have to practice it yourself for some time before you can pass it on to those who have faith in it and have a karmic connection. I met with calamity this time, but fortunately the protector spirits looked over me and I escaped death. During this convalescence period, I felt I shouldn't let my body sit idly for too long, which would affect the movement of my *qi* and blood. Consequently, I remembered when I was young, on a mountain with a Daoist elder who imparted this *daoyin* technique and key training points to me. Revising these techniques after my illness, I found them to be extremely effective in speeding up my recovery. If you intend to learn them, I will perform them a few more times and you can observe closely, in order to remember them well." After *sifu* had given these instructions, he strolled over to an empty space in the courtyard and, in a voice bright and clear, gave out the oral instructions in song form. At this point, clusters of students started making their way into *sifu*'s residence. After they had greeted him one by one with clasped hands, they found places to stand by the sides.

Sifu sang: "First, find a location with good airflow that isn't busy or noisy, which makes it ideal to practice this set—it is very simple and suitable for modern people. Spend a few minutes doing it every day and you can receive tremendous benefits. Begin by standing and adjusting your breath, one to seven times, relaxing your entire body. Next, imagine a sensation of warmth on the *yongquan* points of the soles of both feet. Very lightly, focus your attention there and bend your knees without going past the toes. Your arms then gently and effortlessly float up to the level of the *tanzhong*, shaped as if you were embracing a tree. From here, adjust the breath until you feel comfortable. Breathe in and out 21 times. When inhaling, the tongue curls up to the palate behind the top teeth. When exhaling, the tongue sits in the lower jaw. Repeat this motion with every breath.

Having finished the breathing preparation, slowly return the body to the original standing position, with your arms to the sides of the thighs. Move the arms up the sides to the height of the shoulders, inhaling slowly as you do so; then the arms cross in front of the chest, gathering inward. Continue moving the arms toward the body as if hugging yourself. The palms slap behind the shoulders, then return to the original position, exhaling as they do so. Do this 7 to 21 times. An important note when doing any of the exercises in this set is to pay attention that during the inhalation, the tongue rolls up, and during the exhalation, it rolls downward. When inhaling, lift the *huiyin* (perineum) slightly, as the soles of the feet grip the ground very lightly, but the entire body must be thoroughly relaxed; there cannot be any tension or contraction of the muscles. As you exhale, the soles of the feet and the *huiyin* both relax.

In the second exercise, bend the knees and swing the arms. Following the previous exercise, continue to swing the arms in the same way, only this time, when the arms cross, both knees go from the previous standing posture to a crouching one. Don't bend the knees past the tips of the toes. When crouching down, inhale; when returning to standing, exhale. Repeat this exercise 7 to 21 times, making sure to coordinate the movement with the breath.

In the third form, stand and swing the upper body. Coordinate the arms, swinging them to and fro like a rattle drum. Slap behind the shoulder and along the side of the waist. If the upper half of the body is going left, the palm of the right hand hits the side of the left shoulder, and the left palm slaps the right side of the waist, and vice-versa when turning the other way. Repeat this action 7 to 21 times. When the upper body is twisting, the head and the arms move in unison with it. The breath is natural. This exercise does not require you to focus on the tip of the tongue, the soles of the feet, or the *huiyin*; keep them all naturally relaxed.

In the fourth exercise, cross the two hands as if they were a *taiji* symbol, and place them on the *dantian*. Press on the abdomen and rub in a circular, clockwise motion 36 times. After that, rub in the opposite direction 36 times. Then inhale, pressing the tongue up to the palate, and stand on your toes. When lifting onto the toes, the hands raise over the head, palms facing up; then separate the hands as you exhale, and let the arms float downward, like a bird adducting its wings back toward the body. Concurrently, the heels settle back to the ground. This counts as one repetition. Repeat the practice a total of 7 to 21 times.

For the fifth exercise, clap the hands together and rub them, imagining a hot, burning ball of fire on each *laogong* point on the palms, like a bright sun. Repeat the clapping and rubbing three times. Once the hands are hot, place them on the forehead, cheeks, and the back of the head to warm these areas. Then clap the hands and rub them again as before. When they are hot, rub the chest and then the kidney area. In the same way, rub your body from the chest and back, down to the inner thighs, glutes, hamstrings, and calves, all the way down until you feel comfortable.

In the sixth form, the feet are shoulder-width apart. Breathe naturally, then lean the upper body back. As you lean back, the two arms follow the motion and open backward. Then, as the upper body returns to the vertical, the arms open upward, then continue moving forward, as the upper body bows down. Inhale when leaning backward, exhale when moving forward and down. Repeat this exercise 7 times.

For the seventh exercise, the feet are again shoulder-width apart, with the hands on top of each other, palms facing up, in front of the *dantian*. First regulate the breath 3 to 7 times, then, inhaling slowly, gradually move the hands up to the *tanzhong* in the middle of the chest. As the inhalation fills the chest, stick it out; then the arms push forward and open to the sides, as if gliding on water, as you exhale smoothly. The body then bends forward, bending at the waist as if you were picking something up off the floor, but the knees do not bend. Breathe naturally, as the left and right arm begin to move up and down, vertically, in alternating fashion, a number of times. After this, begin swinging the arms to touch the left leg, then the right leg: your intention is to not use force; rather be completely relaxed, swinging as a rope moving to and fro in the blowing wind. Then return to the arms hanging vertically in front of the legs, move them up and down, then swing them to one side, then the other. Repeat the cycle of the three movements—up and down, to the left, to the right—3 to 7 times. Then return the body to the original standing position, hands over one another in front of the *dantian* as before. Finally, regulate the breath 3 to 7 times.

In the eighth exercise, standing with legs shoulder-width apart, adjust the breath until comfortable and natural. Then put the hands on the hips and do a series of twisting motions with the neck. First, lift the head back, looking up, then move it forward, looking down. Do this 7 times. Then twist and look to the left and right 7 times. Lastly, circle the head around clockwise, then counter-clockwise, moving 360° degrees, a total of 7 times in each direction. Next, the arms rise and stretch out horizontally to the sides; the upper body twists from head to waist, first to the left as far as you are able, and then returns to the original position. Inhale while twisting the upper body, exhale when returning it to the center. Inhale again, this time twisting the upper body to the right, repeating the same action as to the left, again exhaling when returning to the original position. Repeat the twists to the left and right a total of seven times. Then, widen your stance wider than the shoulders. Begin inhaling slowly and squat down, as if you were sitting down on a low wooden bench, all the way until your glutes are parallel with your knees. Exhale as you smoothly rise back up to standing. Repeat this squatting motion 7 to 21 times.

For the ninth exercise, adjust the breath until comfortable. Just like in the fifth exercise, clap the hands together and rub them until hot, then place them over the kidneys and rub in a circular motion 36 times. Clap the hands again and rub them until hot, then massage the buttocks, the inner thighs, the outer thighs, and down to the calves. Finally, sit on the floor, clap and rub the hands together until hot again, 3 times, then massage the bottom of the feet and the *yongquan* points, and use the thumbs to massage the area in between the metatarsals, especially pressing the acupoints there, pushing out toward the toes. Don't use too much force to press outward—use a comfortable amount of pressure.

In the tenth form, place the feet shoulder-width apart and

regulate the breath until natural and comfortable. Visualize the entire sky above of an azure blue, cloudless and clear. The air is full of the five elements of the universe, in the five colors, which come together as in a rainbow. As you inhale, visualize all the auspicious *qi* of the five colors between Heaven and Earth converging; and as you breathe in, the *qi* and colors slowly fill your entire body, entering from the crown of the head. As you exhale, imagine all the discomfort inside your body becoming gray smoke, exhaling it out. When you exhale, make a 'HA!' sound while bending the body forward about 90°. Once the exhalation is complete, return to the original posture, and inhale again, repeating the previous cycle 3 to 7 times.

For the eleventh exercise, place the feet shoulder-width apart and regulate the breath until comfortable. As you inhale, slowly raise the hands up, as you stand on your toes lifting the heels off the ground. Continue inhaling as the arms rise to the sides of the head, palms now facing the sky and pressing up with some force. As you press up, the eyes open wide and stare into the void, while you forcefully exhale and make a 'HA' sound, expelling all the turbid *qi* from inside the body through your mouth. Then return to the original stance and repeat the cycle 3 to 7 times.

The twelfth exercise renders the breath natural, and relaxes the body and mind completely. We begin with the movement of the eyeballs: close both eyes and move them left and right 7 to 21 times, then up and down in a 360° circular motion. Next, rub the palms together to generate heat, then use the hands to warm the face, from the forehead down to the chin, massaging the entire face until it is comfortable, at least 7 times. Then clack the teeth together 7 to 36 times, followed by clapping and rubbing the hands together again, and massaging the neck, chest and back, continuing all the way down to the calves, until comfortable. Finally, return to the original position, feet shoulder-width apart, and regulate the breath until smooth and natural."

Sifu very benevolently explained and demonstrated the exercises for the students. He said this set was originally performed on the mountains by Daoist practitioners at the time of their morning and evening meditations, to maintain the health of the physical body. Originally, there were more movements in the sequence, but *sifu* later improved it by simplifying the exercises. Pairing it with breath cultivation and regulation, the set vivifies the bones, muscles, and tendons and prevents stagnation within the eight channels. Meditators in the initial stages can practice this set before or after their sitting meditation. It is beneficial to one's health, helping in cultivating *qi*, regulating the spirit, and replenishing essence to distill it into *qi*.

Sifu continued: "Originally, I would practice morning and night both the exercises in the *Tendon Changing Classic* and in the *Marrow Cleansing Classic*, as well as the longevity methods practiced by mountain dwellers. However, this accident caused some harm to my original *qi*, so for the time being I didn't want to put too much strain on my body. Therefore, I took these practices I learned on the mountain and pieced them into a simplified form of *daoyin* gymnastics. Doing this exercise set during this time period, coupled with my medicinal concoctions, I was able to recover extremely fast. I've used simple colloquial language to explain these exercises to you: in this modern age—it isn't necessary to name every channel and acupoint or to speak in arcane ways no one understands to flaunt your wit. I myself have never cared much for such theatrics. As long as it helps modern people, I feel it should be promoted. If you have an interest in learning it, you can give it a try. What results can one hope for? It depends solely on one's own effort and determination."

The set of exercises explained above was passed down by *sifu* under opportune conditions when the time was ripe. As far as I know, a few of my Daoist co-practitioners still practice this to this day. Back when we were studying this, some were 20 years my senior, yet all those who have kept up the practice appear to be in great mental and physical condition, with a mind free of afflictions, not showing signs of degeneration to the same extent as those of a similar age. If this practice is done persistently, along with meditation and observance of austerities, you will certainly experience unimaginable wonders.

While *sifu* was explaining this set of exercises, he also spoke about the importance of posting practice. *Sifu* stressed that cultivating one's health is an essential component of practice, and that the mind and physical health must be cultivated and improved together. Through their experimentation through successive generations, Daoist masters agree that posting and meditation practice are different tools to achieve the same goal. Particularly, if one can achieve a state of complete and utter relaxation while posting, one will enter into the stage of working with true *qi*. At this point, one's original *qi* can naturally and freely circulate throughout the eight channels and the entire musculoskeletal system. Such an unhindered state has the effect of loosening internal blockages and obstructions. When those with a more sensitive constitution relax and enter stillness, the entire body will be filled with a rippling energy, vigorously undulating from head to toe, to the point of causing trembling. At this time, do not be alarmed. As long as the mind and the brain are both alert and aware of all movements and everything that is taking place, there is nothing to be worried about. This is entirely different from the state of spirit possession one may experience during Taiwanese folk rituals. People who practice posting sincerely and diligently will—even after only a short time of about ten days—observe changes in their entire body. Students new to posting practice will feel their body change from weak to vigorous, an increase in energy, and improved sleep quality. If the digestive tract is relatively weak, some may also feel an increased appetite. Over time, those who pair posting practice with sitting meditation can open up channels that have been obstructed for half their lifetime.

Speaking of posting, in my early days with *sifu*, as I was leading an elementary meditation and *qigong* class, one of the students who was sitting in the lotus posture suddenly started shaking to the point he was bouncing up and down on his cushion. When *sifu* saw this, he casually walked up to him and quietly whispered some words into his ear. The student's shaking stopped as suddenly as it had started, and he became still. During a short break between sessions, *sifu* addressed those in attendance, saying: "The reason this fellow practitioner was uncontrollably trembling and jumping just now is simply a reflex prompted by the abundance of energy bustling in his body. Since his state of mind then was very clear, all I had to do was gently whisper to him to place his attention on a certain acupoint, thus solving the matter. When practicing meditation, it is unavoidable to experience certain physiological responses, such as rashes that become itchy and swollen, or aches, numbness, isolated muscular twitches, or trembling. In our friend's case, his internal energy had been cultivated to an extent that caused trembling, but he only needed to either pay it no mind or divert his attention for it to stop."

Anaerobic Disease— Regulate Breath to Benefit Life

If Daoist practitioners and meditators themselves can be somewhat versed in medical knowledge, it will be a great help to their breath regulation and retention, meditation, and *daoyin* practice. For example, other than the previously described physiological reactions, some meditators will also experience vomiting and diarrhea, hiccups and gas, heavy perspiration, and the body becoming swollen and hot. These are natural side effects of breathing practice, meditation, and posting, and should not be a cause for worry.

From a physical and mental health perspective, we need to understand that the appropriate use of breathing techniques is the best medicine. In our lives, there are more and more indescribable mental diseases and cancers. These are our century's common ailments, but the root often comes from a problem with breathing. External and internal breathing must complement each other for our body to be healthy. Modern people's biggest problem is simply that they lack oxygen. The reason is that nature is continually damaged by humans, and as a result each breath we take in contains a large amount of carbon dioxide. If we are constantly exposed to various kinds of oils and smoke in our environment, we are constantly depleting our oxygen. Our body's insufficient supply in oxygen has become a big environmental problem. Modern people's nervous mental states, prolonged time spent immobile in climatized or heated spaces, and lack of cardiovascular exercise, cause our emotions to be unstable and make us sensitive to ambient anxiety. Even in our sleep our cranial nerves are operating. Long periods in these states naturally leads to oxygen deficiency. If you don't have the simple methods of sitting meditation or posting to replenish yourself, you will obviously feel that, come the evening, although you want to be active you simply lack the strength, your eyes will be hazy, and you might have chronic headaches, dizziness, nausea, and vomiting. Actually, if you have studied meditation, you will be aware that these mental and physical responses find cause in the excessive waste of oxygen and inability to replenish it quickly.

The most important thing for humans on Earth is oxygen. If we are constantly immersed in an environment poor in oxygen, the amount of carcinogens is likely to increase immensely. Our diet is also an important factor. In the 1920s, the Americans invented refrigeration, which later spread across the globe. People became accustomed to keeping their leftovers in the fridge. Actually, frozen food can have a negative effect on the body. Western countries during the last several decades have also quickly developed many kinds of electric appliances to make cooking more convenient for modern people. But in reality, the food that is cooked with radiation and magnetic waves later passes through our mouth, esophagus, and stomach, and once inside our body, is transformed into many kinds of substances that harm our organs and viscera. Furthermore, there is a plethora of foods replete with artificial preservatives and dyes, chemicals used to make food look more appealing and to lengthen its shelf-life for convenience—modern technology being used to enhance color, fragrance, and taste un-naturally. If there is not enough oxygen in the body to properly metabolize these substances passing through the body, then they will do great harm to our body. Modern people may have mental trouble, perhaps overexerting themselves mentally and physically, under a ton of pressure, and many people use eating as a reliable way to de-stress. A great number of people are overweight, over-burdening the kidneys and giving rise to blood sugar problems and other pathologies.

If the food you eat for your three meals is more than your body needs, then free radicals can be constantly created. The result of technological development, although convenient for modern people, and also providing a more comfortable experience, does not entirely understand protecting the human body, and so we spend long amounts of time exposed to heated or cooled rooms while doing activities. From maps of the entire world, you can see the distribution: countries in tropical regions and those that use geothermal or centralized heating for long periods have higher levels of hypoxia compared to other countries. If we are under a lot of psychological stress for a long period without regular alleviation, it will cause our mind and body great harm, and can create an anaerobic response in the body. Modern people have gradually developed awareness of a health crisis. Therefore, many people take time to run or to stretch, do gymnastics, yoga, or various other kinds of activities for their body to keep fit. If the heart organ function hasn't reached a healthy standard value for a long time, there is a chance for hypoxia in the body to increase. You can exercise and sweat every day, which will increase the heart pulse strength, and is also a great help to your health. Moreover, if before going to the hospital for a health check-up, your body regularly has a sense of idiopathic aches and pains or sleeplessness, if you yawn frequently, easily feel dizzy or have headaches, nausea, and vomiting, a likely diagnosis is hypoxia.

During the last couple of years, I have heard of a number of people I know passing away in their sleep, and of more who work overtime and overburden their bodies, suddenly dropping dead. These people, for the most part, were elite members of society, and simply did not have the time to exercise and sweat, possibly irritating the heart, which, coupled with the weight of their psychological stress, quickly depleted their internal oxygen. Over time this causes irreversible pathologies to arise within the body. Therefore, if you yourself on a regular basis feel dizzy for no apparent reason and are unable to concentrate, along with prolonged stifling pain in the chest, if you regularly snore during sleep, and experience long bouts of sore or hoarse throat, of allergies or itchy rashes, all these symptoms are actually related to a prolonged state of myocardial hypoxia. Many people seek to find the causes that are the reason for their body's allergies, but are unable to come up with a diagnosis. This is because all these problems lie in deep-seated psychological stress. If our body is constantly subjugated to a hypoxic state, this can lead to damage to the body's cells. If a particular area of cells is frequently damaged, that area becomes highly prone to developing cancer. Therefore, finding a way to allow cells to directly acquire oxygen—especially highly active oxygen—is a subject very much worth researching. The reason why the human body has inflammation problems is also due to a loss of antioxidant ability. Over time, free radicals can directly cause harm to our cells. This can give rise to inflammation, or can possibly cause a negative change to our genes.

Thus, the person who understands meditation should have a fundamental concept about staying healthy. Don't disregard your body, as this is inverting the root and the fruit. If the physical body has not attained a basic standard of health, and in addition it is in an environment lacking proper oxygen, then even if you meditate every day, the result will not be very good. If you do seated meditation for a long time, you know how to relieve the stress and emotions of your mind, have healthy habits, keep an appropriate diet, and your mind doesn't give rise to any kind of negative thinking. There are telltale signs on your face and body. For instance, unlike people who do not regularly practice meditation, you don't easily develop wrinkles or age spots, or any forms of pigmentation on the skin, and your muscles and joints don't easily get inflamed.

If in your own meditation practice you haven't yet reached the stage where dreaming and waking are of one taste (i.e., one and the same), it's imperative that your body and mind get sufficient rest. I once knew a lay practitioner in Taichung who was mainly self-taught. It was said that since he was young he practiced meditation and *qi*-refinement. Perhaps due to karma from a past life, his meditation had allowed him the ability to help others by using *qi* to treat illnesses. I once advised him that if his physical body had not yet been completely purified, he should avoid as much as possible giving others his painstakingly acquired true *qi*. This is especially true in the case of illness, because the cause of the patient's sickness can have implications: that is, if it comes from a karmic debt or obstacle. This is analogous to someone with debts pushing back payment: the creditors will naturally come forth to claim what is their due. However, if you forcefully intervene and make a mess of the accounts, will the creditors just peacefully let matters rest? Other than illness which comes from naturally induced imbalances, a plethora of diseases and discomforts are related to the karma of past lives. If cultivators are unclear about cause and effect, or even conceal it through misguided compassion, they will cause of obstacles for themselves. My Daoist friend in Taichung was overconfident in his *qigong* ability, and treated people every day through *qi* emission. One day, while chatting over a meal, he said he felt dizzy and went to the restroom. While in there, he collapsed and was discovered by some of the restaurant staff, who then called an ambulance. He passed away en route to the hospital. He was not yet 50 years old. I have seen and heard of these kinds of matters happening many times over the years. Although you shouldn't practice selfishly, before you have achieved the Great Dao, you should cultivate your own self and practice within your capacity.

CHAPTER 19

THE FIRST STEP TO CULTIVATING HEALTH— UNITING BREATH AND MIND

One day, I came across these words of advice, which I believe could bring great assistance to any practitioner in their daily cultivation: "Don't ponder over good and evil; let the inhale and exhale go without a trace; lend often your ear to observe and listen pointedly to emptiness; silently veil your eyes and observe finely." When your skill in meditation matures, you will start to realize that, to truly adjust the breath, there can be no separation from stillness and movement, from day and night. Generally speaking, an individual will take an average of at least 14,000 breaths a day. If they can truly meld their mind and breath, be perfectly clear of every distinct moment, and turn their gaze toward their unconcealed self-nature when silent, in time it will become possible for them to concentrate their focus on their acupoints and understand the principle of the correspondence between the mind and the breath.

Among the venerable elders I had the chance to call upon, almost all invariably kept the topic of conversation to methods pertaining to regulating the breath and cultivating health. At the stage of gathering the medicine in particular, having sufficient physical energy and getting enough sleep are rather important. One day, while I was studying meditation at *sifu*'s home, he taught some sitting and sleeping methods of the Luo Sect. According to the elders, before you have attained fruition in your practice, cultivating and protecting the liver and kidneys is extremely important. If the quality of your sleep is poor, you will have insufficient kidney *qi*, and will have no way of producing *yang qi*. If your sleep is disturbed by many dreams, thoughts, and restlessness, you will be unable to collect your spirit and retain your *qi*, and you will have no hope of harmonizing your fire and water *qi*. One elder said something even more fascinating: "The mark of your cultivation of the Dao is how well you sleep. Thus, it is said that the accomplished true man neither dreams nor worries." I think there is a lot of sense in these words.

Regardless of whether you are entering meditation or sleep, you must invariably put all considerations aside, focus on your mind, and finely adjust your breath. Place your attention gently on the *dantian*, unite the essence, *qi* and spirit, and by no means let the spirit drift outward. With the mind and breath in perfect unison, naturally allow yourself to enter sleep. *Sifu* once said: "The Luo Sect has its own set of sleep practices. The head must be facing East. Incline the body and rest on the side, in the way a dog would. Bend one arm under your head to serve as a pillow and with the other rub your *dantian* region in a circular motion 36 times. Before your massage, you must first suggest to yourself to forget about all things past, present, and future. Once this preparation is done, you can close your eyes. One leg is outstretched and the other is folded. Breathe in and out naturally." *Sifu* shared that, after sleeping in this way for a time, his spirit and *qi* felt bright and invigorated. He was astonished by the effects.

Although the great medical scholar of the Song Dynasty, Yang Renzhai, evolved as a medical practitioner in an ordinary traditional rural setting, he developed outstanding proficiency and produced a stack of writings as tall as himself. In due time, word spread and he became regarded as one of the "three great doctors of the Song." The *materia medica* he gathered and compiled in his *Effective Recipes from the Renzhai House* is to this day highly esteemed in the world of Traditional Chinese Medicine and is still used as reference material.

To get to the heart of the matter, Yang Renzhai had a keen interest in Buddhism, Daoism, and Confucianism, and extensively perused their respective literature. Moreover, he practiced breath regulation exercises daily. That is why in such an early date in history, he was able to postulate that the circulation of *qi* and blood is the main factor in recovering from illness. He advocated that the best way to cure disease was to cultivate and harmonize both circulatory systems.

His contribution to medical science is not limited to this. Indeed, as early as the Song Dynasty, he mentioned "a growth that protrudes and sinks in, similar to the face of a rock," which is a very clear and unequivocal description of cancer, one of the banes of our times. Therefore, if we can manage to free up a little time in our daily schedule to practice posting and other *daoyin* methods along with breath regulation, and work toward uniting the breath and mind, we will very naturally rid ourselves of any worries concerning the state of our health.

Cheng Tinghua was a very renowned grandmaster of *xingyi* and *bagua*[1] in the early days of the Republic of China. At one point, his fame spread throughout the country among practitioners of internal martial arts. Among all his disciples, Sun Lu Tang was the one who distinguished himself the most in his teacher's eyes, and, indeed, he lived up to the latter's expectations and founded the Sun style of *taiji*. When Xu Shijing became President, he sent a personal invitation to Sun Lu Tang to be a military attaché in his government. Moreover, Sun Lu Tang achieved a certain renown overseas, notably by defeating fighters representing the Japanese Emperor and knocking Russian fighters out cold. The Japanese remained thoroughly unconvinced by his performance and sent five more elite fighters in the hopes of making him capitulate. Sun Lu Tang brought their bravado to a swift and definite end, and his heroism was spoken of widely.

I once listened to my teacher speak of the times in which Sun Lu Tang lived, and how the master had once crossed paths with

---

1   八卦 or 八卦掌 (*baguazhang*): One of the three main (internal) martial arts of the Wudang style, the other two being *taiji* and *xingyi*.

another famous internal martial arts master, a man who was highly skilled in *baguazhang* and who had also been a disciple of Cheng Tinghua. His feet and palm movements were too fast for the eye to catch, like a flash of lightning, and his stride was as fast and formless as the wind. At one time he occupied the post of martial arts instructor at the Central Guoshu Institute, and *sifu* said that his particularity was the way he combined the posting methods of *bagua* and *xingyi* with breathing methods in instructing his disciples. As a matter of fact, the results were incredible, and they noticed great progress in both formless practice and martial forms and stances. He went even further and started popularizing posting and breath regulation among the masses, allowing it to become a rather common practice at the time, and it is said that he also helped many people sort out long-standing chronic ailments and diseases that were deemed incurable. The *qigong* and breath regulation methods he taught were, moreover, exceedingly simple, and consisted essentially of meditation and posting. People who had physical disabilities could practice breath regulation lying down. He advocated letting the in-breath and out-breath come and go naturally, and distinguished various types of breath, from shallow to deep. If you look carefully at his *qigong* instructions, you will find that they don't depart much from what Daoism consistently teaches. What we can understand from this is that, whether you are a martial artist or an athlete, whether you are at rest or in motion, the most important thing is to first and foremost enter stillness; then, within this state of stillness, adjust the breath to finally enter a state where the mind and spirit are united, where the mind and breath correspond. If you cultivate and maintain this state, your body will naturally return to its original state of health and serenity.

CHAPTER 20

DOING AWAY WITH INSOMNIA THROUGH MEDITATION AND REGULATION OF THE MIND

During *sifu*'s demonstration of these health cultivation methods that day, some more elderly fellow practitioners present asked some questions concerning sleep. Among them was Mr. Huang, who was in his early sixties at the time. He had been meditating for over 20 years by then, but for some cause unknown to him, in that period of time he had trouble sleeping. Every night, he would toss and turn countless times, troubled and restless. Seeing that the topic of sleep had been brought up, Mr. Huang seized the opportunity to consult *sifu* about his problem.

Sifu nodded and explained: "From the perspective of Chinese Medicine, poor quality of sleep is due to the *yang* channels being too exuberant. This makes the body unable to regulate the five organs, which in turn leads to vacuous *yin qi*. One's sleep will thus be poor in quality and there will be a lot of tossing and turning. Another possible cause is related to the *yangqiao* meridian, which branches out from the *taiyang* channel and controls the movement of muscles around the eyes. When it receives signals of sleepiness, it transmits a message to the eyes' nervous system to close and go to sleep. But if the *yinqiao* channel's *yang qi* is overstimulated, you could spend the whole night with your eyes wide open, unable to sleep soundly. If in addition to this, you have no *daoyin* practice routine to adjust any imbalance and your circulation of *qi* and blood declines, your *yin* and *yang* will become inverted.

It is common to see symptoms of an exuberant amount of energy during the day, but due to poor circulation of *qi* and blood across the five organs, the nervous system is too stimulated and it will be difficult to wind down at night and sleep. There are many causes for poor quality of sleep. Older individuals will often have vacuous *yin*, causing insufficiency in blood and essence. This leads to the inability to harmonize one's *yin* and *yang qi*, and hence poor sleep. Vacuous *yin* for the most part comes from psychological factors: excessive happiness, anger, thinking, and sudden and unexpected shocks that cause dejection and grief, or perhaps excessive worry, anxiety, and fear. If you remain in these states of mind for prolonged periods of time without processing or reaching closure, they will cause your liver and kidneys to be out of balance and your sleep will be negatively affected as well. Modern people's social interactions are too numerous, and business obligations and other causes of stress can lead to depletion of the liver's blood and the kidney's *qi*. Over an extended period, this will cause the vacuous fire to be over-exuberant, which then leads to excessive worry and unstable emotions, and thus poor sleep. For cultivators of the Daoist path, the three treasures of essence, *qi*, and spirit are paramount. If you're unable to settle down your spirit, how can you hope for sound sleep? Those who overthink things are especially prone to having negative *qi* enter their body, which will lead to poor blood and *qi*, as well as bad circulation. So, why have I been urging you all from early on to cultivate a meditation practice and an understanding of the *Scripture of Purity and Quiescence*,[1] the *Dao De Jing* and the *Zhuangzi*? Do you understand now?

These classics all explain very clearly how we are to let go of our inner obstacles and attachments, how to remain at all times in a natural and pure state of mind, characterized by non-action. Couple this with your meditation practice until you reach the state of empty, wondrous illumination,[2] and you will naturally enter the

---

1   清靜經 (*qingjingjing*): An anonymous Tang Dynasty Daoist classic on the elimination of desire in order to cultivate spiritual purity and stillness.
2   虛靈妙明 (*xu ling miao ming*): Very generally, a high state of meditative stillness.

state of ultimate purity, emptiness, and illumination,[3] bereft of any disturbance from outside phenomena. If on top of this, you can bear a mind free from desire and pursuits, your mind will become even more peaceful and undistracted. Gradually, the six dusts of forms, sounds, smells, tastes, touch, and thoughts will cease to have an effect on you. In time, whether during the day or at night, your mind will be clear, bright, and discerning. How then could you experience trouble sleeping? You have been meditating for such a long time and yet have not even gone through the process of plucking the medicine. You should ask yourself whether your personal aspirations and desires are perhaps too deep-set? Or perhaps you have accumulated so many habitual patterns that they are too hard to change, resulting in a depressed state? This is really not desirable. I have been reminding you of the importance of the cultivation of character for so many years now. Meditation requires hard work, especially in respect to one's temperament. You must have perseverance, until your mind is totally bereft of fire, smoke, and odor. Only then will you have the prerequisites to refine your essence into *qi*, and your *qi* into spirit, and from there give rise to all things, wherein your life-force is plentiful and your circulation unimpeded. If you sit in these conditions, you will have the chance to practice inner alchemy. All of you must pay very close attention here. You can assess whether or not you have passed the portal of meditation by observing yourselves and asking yourselves a few questions: if you had any illness when you started meditating, did it gradually improve and get better? If you catch a small cold or similar minor ailment, are you quick to recover? Has your immune system and general resistance to disease gotten stronger? Are your internal organs and viscera operating smoothly? Do you have any ailments brought about by vacuous fire in your internal organs?

At the very least, you must be able to ensure that no disease will be bred inside you, nor any virus invade you from the outside. Only after achieving this can we start to discuss how to avoid getting

---

3　太清, 太虛, 太明 (*taiqing, taixu, taiming*): Also, a high state of meditative stillness.

old, how your fallen teeth and hair can regrow through meditation and how to have very fine, lustrous, and flawless skin, etc. On the surface, you all say you are meditating, yet your minds are running around, delusive thoughts swirling all over, and however hard you try, you are unable to settle down. How can this be considered stillness? And if you are unable to settle in stillness, how can you reach quietude? In meditation, if you are unable to enter quietude, your practice will not bear fruit. Meditation itself is actually removed from awakening, or enlightenment, by a very long shot. Be that as it may, you must at the very least, first cultivate emptiness and unify yourself with the Dao. Only then will you be accomplishing the dual practice of body and mind, and only then do you have a hope of longevity. Other complementary *daoyin* methods such as posting are extremely helpful to the health and well-being of the physical body, but they remain a great distance away from awakening to the Dao."

Sifu very placidly and tolerantly led this senior student and others present through the steps, and very candidly provided them with his own understanding. Yet, out of fear that those in attendance might have misunderstood, he went on to explain in plainer words: "To be honest, in the long time I've been in Taiwan I've come across countless people suffering with insomnia. Modern medicine generally recommends people should get seven to eight hours of sleep a night, but sleeping excessively is also not a good sign. In Western countries, these are referred to as sleep disorders, and when looked into closely do not differ much from the Chinese medical perspective. Generally speaking, these obstacles rarely depart much from the physical and mental duress that the struggles of daily life bring upon people. Thinking too much will inevitably cause you to be ill-at-ease, whether sitting or standing, and unable to sleep soundly. For some people, this is due to the great deal of nervousness and anxiety they experience during the day, which translates into insomnia come night time. For others, it is caused by the ingestion of stimulating foods that harm their gastrointestinal system and deny them restful sleep. Regardless, such problems mostly find root in physiological factors. Some people also experience these difficulties due to spatio-temporal factors such as time changes, or sudden changes in their daily schedule or in their environment, but if you understand how to meditate and regulate your breath, these problems can be solved easily."

CHAPTER 21

THE INTERCOMMUNICATION OF THE THREE DOCTRINES

In my earlier years studying Daoist alchemy under my master, I heard about how some fellow practitioners, either out of curiosity or simply prompted by friends, took up the practice of Indian yoga. They were scarcely aware that they had gone far away to seek that which was close by. What's more, their sectarian friends did not always speak the truth. One of the reasons I hold the teachings of the School of Complete Reality in high esteem is because a great number of its lineage masters practiced both Daoism and Buddhism, never excluding those who are on a different spiritual path. They have great reverence for Buddhism particularly.

Lineage patriarch Wang Chongyang of the School of Complete Reality went thus far to advocate the trio practices of Confucianism, Buddhism, and Daoism. He demonstrated the imposing grandeur of a remarkable lineage master endowed with penetrating insight that is rare to behold. Inspired by this, while immersing myself in Daoist thought, I once tried to trace back its origin in history to understand how the three schools developed and eventually integrated. I realized that the trajectory of the three schools in China, from Emperor Wu of Liang down to the Yuan, Ming, and Qing dynasties, showed ample precedents of the three supplementing one another. This was particularly common among community organizations throughout the country.

During the reign of Emperor Wu of Liang, Master Tanluan was revered as the most important Pureland School master. Devoting almost his entire life to the propagation of the Pureland School teachings, he nevertheless read a sizeable amount of Daoist classics and received teachings from notable Daoist practitioners during his youth. He was well versed in all three schools—Confucianism, Buddhism, and Daoism—which would prove to be tremendously beneficial when he started to lecture and spread the *dharma* in the future. In the earlier period of his lectures, he provided truly original and insightful discourses on sutras of *Prajna* (wisdom) and *Madhyamaka* (Middle Way). He also annotated copious amounts of important Buddhist sutras.

Due to a karmic connection, Master Tanluan became acquainted with a Daoist practitioner named Tao Hongjing, while seeking a cure for a chronic disease that ailed him. Having been treated successfully by Tao, he learned an extremely secret *qi* cultivating practice from the Daoist sage. After putting the exercise into practice, sure enough, he felt invigorated and full of energy, so much so that it appeared that he was never going to exhaust that energy. It was said that ever since Master Tanluan read the *Amitāyurdhyāna Sūtra*,[1] he decided to devote his life to reciting Amitābha Buddha's name. According to his biographies written by later generations, not only was Master Tanluan a lineage patriarch and prolific Buddhist commentator, he'd also compiled and penned scores of Daoist books on *qi* cultivation and medicine-related subjects. We can thus derive the idea that besides being a Bodhisattva, on the path of reciting the Buddha's name Master Tanluan also put much emphasis on health cultivation.

On the Chan side of the story, before the first patriarch Bodhidharma passed on his lineage to an heir, he'd been poisoned many times. So extremely toxic was the poison that even a rock would break open upon coming into contact with his feces. He used his supernatural power to detoxify the harmful substance to buy time before his heir, the second patriarch, Shenguang, would appear. Shenguang had gone through similar atrocities to his predecessor's: the patriarch of the Tiantai Sect of Buddhism, Master

---

1   Literally, *Amitāyus Meditation Sūtra*. One of the three main sutras of the Pure Land tradition in *Mahāyāna* Buddhism, along with the *Amitābha Sutra* and the *Infinite Life Sutra*.

Huisi, was spiked by non-Buddhists on several occasions. Though he managed to stay alive, the residual toxin left in his body nevertheless posed a threat to both his physical body and his meditation practice to some degree. An accidental encounter with a highly achieved Daoist practitioner who gave him advice on the subject, eventually helped him to clean up the residual toxin so that he could continue spreading the *dharma*.

Of all Master Huisi's writings on Buddhism, many of his expositions on meditative stillness are mixed with the oral tips of Daoist patriarchs. What's more, even the discourses of Master Zhiyi (the founder of the Tiantai Sect) upon the joint practice of *śamatha*[2] and *vipaśyanā*,[3] as well as sitting meditation, are fused with Daoist practices of *daoyin*, massage, and breathing techniques and tips. Other notable Buddhist schools also occasionally produced writings which merged Buddhist, Daoist, and Confucian thought. As long as this is beneficial to the body, mind, and spirit of sentient beings, to their cultivation of health and character, to the blossoming of their wisdom and liberation, it is valuable. The most important thing is that the respective views are expressed in a clear manner rather than as a confused jumble of ideas, so as not to misguide the audience. One has to maintain truthfulness in the contemplation, cultivation, and actualization of one's practice, continuing and upholding the eminent mastery of past sages. Whether it's the sagehood evoked by the Confucian scholars, the Nirvana of Buddhism, or Daoist immortality, the most important thing is not to deviate from the standards of how one interacts with society, one's deportment, and how one handles one's affairs. At the very least, one should follow ethical conduct and contribute valuable deeds and words to society. Parting from the Way and virtue does not accord with the doctrine and principles of spiritual practice. Though we might not be able to entirely comprehend truth and

---

2 From the Pali/Sasnkrit, a Buddhist term meaning "calmness of mind," equivalent to the "meditative stillness" (禪定, *chanding*) of Chan/Zen Buddhism.

3 A Sanskrit term, meaning "insight." One of the two main qualities necessary to be developed through meditative practices, the other being *śamatha*/meditative stillness.

nature or accomplish the dual practice of body and mind, at the very least we ought to adjust ourselves so that we don't deviate, even for a moment, from the mind, the very place where all the myriad Dao derive. When it comes to worldly affairs and spiritual pursuit, it is best to try to neither enter it nor withdraw from it. One step further, strive to achieve the state where there is no opposition of *li* (noumenon) and *shi* (phenomenon). Then, there will be nothing left to be remorseful for in this cycle of life.

CHAPTER 22

The Key Point of the School of Complete Reality—Returning to One's True Self-Nature

When I first started learning meditation, I was constantly reminded by the elders of the benefits that the *Hundred Word Inscription* of the Daoist immortal Lu Chunyang (Lu Dongbin) has on meditation as well as cultivating character. The first phrase, "To cultivate *qi*, keep yourself from frivolous speech; to subdue the mind, act without acting," clearly explains the methods of cultivating essence, *qi*, and spirit. When it comes to confronting the Eight Worldly Winds, wield the sword of wisdom to chop all forms of greed till there are no frivolous thoughts left. Only then, can the practitioner achieve the unity of mind and *qi*, where the breathing becomes soundless and so fine that it does not even exist. Naturally, gradually, the elixir will be made.

To achieve this, practitioners must be vigilant in attending to both their mind and spirit, whether during or after meditation, and never depart from them. Breathing must be in sync with this effort so there are no delusive thoughts; only absolute stillness. The mind is subsequently tamed, body and mind are both still. Only then can one truly start to jointly cultivate one's original essence and spirit, and thus truly cultivate one's *qi*. With the mind and intention thus residing in utmost stillness, one can truly cultivate spirit. After you finish a round of meditation practice, don't let the mind wander away within the six dusts and eight winds. In movement, you can also regulate and unify your breath and mind;

true *qi* will then naturally start revolving, warming up the kidney *qi* and harmonizing the water (kidney) and fire (heart) elements. By driving the *qi* by means of our spirit, we can in the long run form the elixir (*dan*) and our *qi* will be replete. Neither the spirit nor *qi* will spill out, and the spirit will return to its original seat. Then, we will naturally feel like we can gather the medicine, our mind will be bright and clear, we will feel something akin to water boiling between our kidneys, and rolls of thunder in our stomach. Additionally, if we are adept at reading the pulse, we can guide our *qi*, starting at the *weilu* (acupoint near the tailbone) and up past the three gates to the crown, where we will experience the state of "ambrosia permeating Mount Meru." At this point, we can "greet it with our eyes and attend to it with our mind." Needless to say, our five organs and six viscera will be replete, and the successive stages of refining essence into *qi*, *qi* into spirit, and finally to return spirit to emptiness, will naturally occur.

Of course, this requires guidance from a practitioner who not only has immersed themselves in the practice but has also received pith instructions to prevent themselves from going astray. This was originally a secret Daoist teaching that cannot be heard by more than three people at a time. I have come across some rather disordered annotations, which often miss the mark, on small book stalls in the street. The fact that they never somehow cut right to the point is quite unfortunate. Therefore, one should take precautions while consulting commentaries on ancient texts. This is due to the precautionary measures taken by our predecessors, who, out of benevolence, intentionally put words in such a way as to blur the meaning for those who are not supposed to receive these teachings. While learning about Daoist alchemy in the past, we used to jot down the oral tips recited by our teacher, who said explicitly that these tips should not be transmitted without meticulous consideration, in order to avoid calamities in the future.

Meditation is a lifelong commitment, not something you expect to achieve by practicing half-heartedly. Indeed there are many, even among fellow practitioners, who go back and forth between progress and regression in their practice. Some persevered but unfortunately lacked the guidance of a qualified master, so ended up not achieving what they had aspired to achieve. Some learned from non-genuine sources that taught false visualizations, which was a huge waste of time and led to self-harm. I've personally witnessed scores of the latter scenario where the practitioners' *qi* and channels were thrown into total disarray, incurable by medicine. It was a very pitiful situation. When it comes to meditation, if you insist on practicing alone but wish to avoid going astray, then you shouldn't cling to the so-called "methods that promise results." The name "Complete Reality" denotes a complete abandoning of physical and mental attachments, thus returning to a state of one's true self where desires are eliminated and the mind is calm. The ultimate goal is to dedicate oneself to the cultivation of both the physical and the spiritual life, the unity of spirit and *qi*, as well as returning to one's true state.

In modern times, however, such requirements are rare, not to mention the fact the people in this era are less likely to attain the ultimate state of purity and emptiness as their elders. I often notice how some young practitioners struggle with such concerns as food, sleep, and relationships. How can we go on to discuss more advanced Daoist alchemy practices? Therefore, while practicing meditation, whether you are sitting on a cushion or getting up from it, moving or not moving, it's essential to remove all the frivolous thoughts in your mind. If they are not removed, the practitioner can never achieve stillness. Likewise, when stillness is achieved and no frivolous thoughts exist, the cultivator can perceive the will of the Heavens. For those who have some meditation experience, it is beneficial to post for five to ten minutes prior to sitting. This will regulate the breath and deeply relax the body and mind, so that the *qi* flows unobstructed.

While sitting, first regulate the breath until both the mind and body are still, before lowering the eyelids. Following that, focus on the *dantian* and make sure the breathing is long and well-paced, as if everything around you is in complete silence and only the breath can be heard. This is true stillness. While breathing, make sure that the breath remains in the space between the heart and kidneys, and that the breath comes in and out smoothly. Continuing this way, the practitioner will gradually notice the *dantian* is getting warmer, as are the kidneys. Subsequently, practitioners will enter the stage of "turtle breathing," where one lets go of the regular way of breathing through in-breath and exhalation. When practitioners achieve this stage, they will discover that their "breath" clearly ceases to go in and out of the nose, a phenomenon called "returning to the root and reviving one's life"[1] in the Daoist world. One step further and practitioners' true *qi* will spontaneously form and start rising vertebra by vertebra from the tail bone upward. Once it reaches the *baihui* (acupoint located at the top of the head), it moves down past the *queqiao* (at the bridge of the nose, between the nostrils) and the *tanzhong* (acupoint located in the center of the chest), finally sinking down into the *dantian* again. Ordinary practitioners will feel overjoyed about reaching this stage, but caution should be exercised as this is not the real opening of one's pathways. It's better not to pay attention to it. When it does occur, there's only one thing to do: neither invite nor reject it. Allow it to move uninterruptedly, but slightly contained. Wait until the spirit, *qi*, and blood are abundant, a stage that needs to be carefully observed for three to six months. When the opportunity becomes ripe, those with the highest level of skill will notice a vigorous quality to their spirit, while true *qi* fills up and starts to surge along the time-tested pathways of the movements of the celestial chariot, a point of practice based on the completion of other stages, such as the "hundred days of building the foundation [through abstinence]," "gathering and obtaining the pill," and the "nine rotations."

---

1   歸根復命 (*guigenfuming*).

CHAPTER 23

LENG QIAN—AN EXEMPLARY IMMORTAL

Many people place both practitioners of the Dao and its accomplished immortals on a cloud, whereas the poems and essays of China depict them quite aptly as beings roaming the empty sky, caressing the clouds with the tips of their fingers and going about life unburdened and at ease. Because of the influence of the various forms of literature, fortune-telling, and rites that are the foundation of their culture, the Chinese people are quite reverential toward the spirit realm. In the vast historical annals of China, such as Mr. Lu's *Spring and Autumn Annals* or *Records of the Grand Historian*, it is common to find reference to the marvels accomplished by immortals. Even Confucius, who had guarded his disciples against discussing spirits and extraordinary powers during the course of their daily lives, taught that they should be reverential of these things and live according to the mandate of Heaven; and *The Analects* itself contains many chapters that discuss topics related to spirits. We can thus see that Chinese culture is inextricably entwined with the ideas of Heaven, Earth, and the gods. In fact, the *Record of the Grand Historian* reveals to us that even the cruel Emperor Qin Shihuang, whose violent rule was marked by auto-da-fé and a war against Confucianism, secretly sent emissaries in search of the elixir of longevity. After the system of thought that saw the three great religions of China as being one complementary whole became commonplace, many scholars and erudite people wantonly pursued the dual practice of Buddhism and Daoism and tried to establish common ground between the two. In the Emperor's palace there were even astronomers who would observe astronomical phenomena and, in partnership with masters of the *Yi Jing* who observed seasons, would make divinations as to the auspicious or inauspicious nature of the omens. The reverence and tribute offered to the spirit realm was thousandfold among the masses. From here on out, Daoist literature and books on Daoist internal alchemy became widespread. Among all the reference works available then, the richest was Ge Hong's *Baopuzi*. As a result of this torrent of intellectual activity, a great number of concise biographies of Daoist immortals was to be found in the Imperial Palace as well as among the people. Even the Confucian tradition was undergoing a silent transformation, and its scholars would seamlessly employ very evocative, romantic, and colorful wording, as well as flights of the imagination to give life to the immortals in their writings, such as this piece by Zhuangzi:

> Far away on the mountain of Gu Ye there dwelt a solitary man, an otherworldly man whose flesh and skin were as ice and snow, his manner as pure as that of a virgin's. He did not eat any of the five grains, but subsisted on the wind and dew; he mounted on the clouds, rode along the flying dragons, rambling and enjoying himself beyond the four seas.

The reason Zhuangzi's *Leisurely Roam* was recorded as an important text of Daoism is due to the mental imagery and character expressive of the immortals. Zhuangzi very wisely makes use of the phrase "forgetting both subject and object," the "object'" an analogy for these two melding together, as a way to elaborate on the "three nothingnesses."[1] The whole essay will invariably leave the reader somewhat perplexed as to the meaning, but at that time it was a thoroughly innovative way of admonishing his readership. Besides, his prose warrants no shackle or limitation; it is formidable and unruly, majestic and uninhibited, of a timeless beauty and elegance.

---

1   三無 (*sanwu*): Namely, no thought, no abiding, and no phenomenon.

CHAPTER 24

NOURISH THE KIDNEYS AND CALM THE MIND—WATER AND FIRE WILL HARMONIZE

I first heard of the "Sixteen Gold Ingots" oral tips from three of my Daoist masters, one of them being my root master, who taught them to me in person. At the time, there were eight of us who received them, and *sifu* said to us: "Just so you know, I don't usually impart these oral tips easily. Daoist master Leng Qian states: 'One inhalation facilitates rising; cycle the breath, return to the navel; one rise facilitates gulping; water and fire thus meet.' If you can put the tips into practice and supplement them with meditation, inner alchemy, you'll surely yield amazing results from the practice. Countless Daoist practitioners have achieved longevity and youthful appearance by practicing this way. One should never take it lightly. I myself practice diligently on a daily basis and consequently I am free from the usual headaches, fevers, and other minor ailments most people suffer from.

Previously I gave a brief introduction to some of your fellow practitioners. What you need to take note of is this: I've met someone who learned the oral tips from elsewhere and seemed to overly stress the part that involves lifting the anus. In actuality, you only need to use the intention to gently lift the anus and you must by all means avoid applying force. Failing to do so might bring about health issues such as hemorrhoids. The 'Sixteen Gold Ingots' oral tips are essentially a set of breathing practices collated by Master Leng Qian after having spent his whole life cultivating health and general well-being. It is a method that helps nourish the kidneys through the symbiotic balance of water and fire.[1] Most people associate the kidneys primarily with sexual functions. In fact, kidneys are more than that. Those with even the slightest knowledge will tell you that our emotions are directly related with our internal organs. The kidneys, for instance, are closely related to one's thoughts. When we are overly nervous, scared, anxious, or worried, our kidneys are harmed.

Being overly anxious will deplete one's kidney *qi*, which results in people indulging in negative emotions or pessimistic thinking. Naturally, when it comes to decision making, they find it hard to make the best judgement. If we follow the Western Medicine principle, this can be explained as being under the influence of adrenaline that leads to the outpouring of various emotions, such as anxiety, depression, etc. Therefore, maintaining a positive mindset, being open-minded, and finding time to relax both the body and mind can directly aid kidney functions. All medicines are relatively toxic, be they Western or Chinese medicines. Unless it's absolutely necessary, one should try to avoid them at all cost. In addition, excessive work and worries can also lead to kidney-related side effects. For instance, a lot of people can't meditate for even ten minutes. Feeling discomfort, they constantly rub their lower backs. This is because they have kidney deficiency,[2] and with the lack of *yang qi*, their blood circulation is unlikely to be in a good condition. In a more serious scenario, lacking appropriate dietary supplements, many people will age prematurely—men experience low libido, wrinkled skin, and hair loss, whereas premature menopause, an unstable emotional state, difficult sleep, and cold sweats will manifest in their female counterparts.

---

1   水火相濟 (*shui huo xiang ji*): The heart is represented by fire and the kidneys by water. These two opposing forces regulate each other in the body; the water (*yang qi*) of the kidneys rises, nourishing the fire (*yin qi*) of heart; the fire of the heart ensures the water element of the kidneys does not get out of control, signifying the balance of *yin* and *yang*.

2   腎水不足 (*shen shui bu zu*): Each organ has its own particular balance of *yin/yang*; any deviation from this balance means the organ is not functioning optimally and this may lead to discomfort.

Chinese Medicine places great emphasis on the correlation between the kidneys and bones. Thus, it's of utmost importance to obtain sufficient calcium from one's diet to avoid osteoporosis. In terms of meditation, the kidneys are directly related to one's essence and *qi*; their importance is demonstrated by the fact that they take up two of the three treasures (the other being spirit). In reality, the kidneys are also related to detoxification, particularly in the form of internal secretion; therefore, the endocrine system is also included in the realm of kidney functions.[3] If you suffer from long-term lower back pain or if the urine is muddy in color, bubbles in the urine do not dissipate immediately, or even blood is found in the urine, then you should definitely seek medical help since these signs indicate that the problem isn't simply deficiency in kidney water.

Thinking that because Chinese Medicine and Daoist practice share the same origin, many Daoist practitioners tend to take Chinese medicine without proper consultation. The fact is, if one fails to fully understand the properties in the medicine and take it long-term, it can actually be harmful to one's kidney function. It can even affect one's daily activities and lead to tumors, which may result, even in the least serious cases, in having to undergo dialysis treatment." These are some basic concepts of Chinese Medicine that *sifu* mentioned in passing one day while while lecturing.

The so-called regulation of "water and fire" in the "Sixteen Gold Ingots" oral tips is essentially about how to utilize the water element in the kidney system to regulate the fire element in the heart system through specific breathing techniques in order to mutually nourish both systems. The saliva produced from the exercise and the moving of *qi* inside the body consists of abundant enzymes and all kinds of beneficial trace elements. Through the regulation of breathing and visualization, one can, over time, avoid and prevent any illnesses caused by the deficiency of *qi* and blood. This includes

---

3   腎臟 (*shenzang*): Contrasted with Western Medicine, the organs in Traditional Chinese Medicine refer not only to the specific organ but to a larger group of functions.

all the wind symptoms[4] related to the nervous system. Regular practice of the "Sixteen Gold Ingots" and "Eight Pieces of Brocade" before and after meditation can definitely be beneficial and supplementary to the improvement of one's meditation practice.

4　風症 (*fengzheng*): Pathologies relating to an imbalance of the wind element in the body (e.g., stroke, bell's palsy, etc.).

CHAPTER 25

THE "EIGHT PIECES OF BROCADE" TO BENEFIT HEALTH AND LONGEVITY

During the process of learning meditation, respectable Daoist teachers transmitted to me countless precious *daoyin* exercises. The goal of *daoyin* practice is not only meditation, guarding the acupoints,[1] and cultivating the *dantian*, but also using the ancient teachings of the immortals preserved in the lineage to support the circulation of the *qi* and blood, clear the channels, and prevent any blood clots from forming. From this panoply of exercises, the "Eight Pieces of Brocade" is particularly revered for its simplicity and effectiveness. This set of exercises is extremely useful for practitioners who either have been meditating for a while, or are observing the no-lying-down precept. The exercises are especially useful for those at an advanced age, whose muscles and bones are likely to lack strength and density. Another benefit of the "Eight Brocades" is that they will activate the 12 main energy channels in the body.[2] These channels pass many hundreds of related acupoints which influence *qi* and blood circulation, regulation of the balance between *yin* and *yang*, and the connective areas between muscles and bones. For most people, a blockage of *qi* can lead to a great number of illnesses, and if there is a failure to understand the

---

1   守竅 (*shouqiao*): The practice of placing one's concentration on various *guanqiao*, or points on the body connected to the Chinese Medicine/Daoist system of meridians and channels.

2   These are: the greater *yin* lung, *yang* brightness large intestine, *yang* brightness stomach, greater *yin* spleen, lesser *yin* heart, greater *yang* small intestine, greater *yang* bladder, lesser *yin* kidney, reverting *yin* pericardium, lesser *yang* triple burner, lesser *yang* gallbladder, and the reverting *yin* liver channel.

underlying reasons, these health issues become chronic. *Daoyin* practitioners need to be particularly careful in order to avoid causing themselves more problems through their practice.

I once asked *sifu*: "What does this elegant name 'Eight Pieces of Brocade' mean?"

He replied: "When I was young, I often saw Daoist priests practicing this up in the mountains, although at that time I didn't give much thought to its lineage and the reasons for doing it. One time Li Qingyun's heart disciple was teaching an English doctor, and only when the Englishman asked about the practice did I begin to understand. Most Daoist schools agree that the practice lineage originated with its transmission by Zhong Liquan, one of the Eight Immortals. However, later on I came across a text from the Ming Dynasty by the Daoist master Leng Qian which did not go so far as to say this, so I'm inclined to think that it's likely just myth and legend, rather than trustworthy fact. Furthermore, the practice of the 'Eight Pieces' began in the Tang Dynasty (618–907). Regarding the many literary works concerning the *dantian*, channels, and other health-promoting practices, all the schools use different abridged and extended versions of these methods; thus, I myself have learned no less than five or six versions. This being said, the beneficial effects are beyond doubt, in regard to the channels and acupoints of the whole body. As for the origins of the name, there are various contrasting explanations, but the one I have heard most often maintains that because the practice involves the channels (*jing*) and the clearance of any obstructions in them to allow a freer flow, the similar sounding word for 'brocade' (*jin*) was picked. Ever since ancient times, this practice has been used by many—not only Daoist practitioners, but also scholars who made it part of their exercise routine in order to protect their health and promote longevity. Its use can be traced back to ancient scholars such as Ouyang Xiu (a Northern Song Dynasty prose writer and historian, 1007–1072) and Su Dongpo (writer and calligrapher, 1037–1101), and even Zhu Xi, as well as other erudite people. Almost all of them were very proficient in using this method.

From a young age I also made it part of my daily routine. If you were to ask me whether I have any concrete proof of its effectiveness, I would recount the time after a traffic accident I had. Someone at my advanced age would usually have to endure hospital stays and possibly operations, let alone after experiencing a serious injury. Nevertheless, for one and a half years after the accident, I consistently prepared my own herbal medicines and nursed myself back to health. Once I could move my limbs again, I resumed my daily practice of the 'Eight Brocades,' the 'Sixteen Brocades,' and the 'Sixteen Gold Ingots,' as well as the various martial arts *taiji* posting methods transmitted to me by other Daoist elders. Strangely, I recovered so rapidly that even I felt such a turnaround was barely believable! I don't wish to give too mystical an elaboration beyond this. Last year, didn't Zhang Yazi's husband suffer a stroke? The doctor said it would be extremely difficult to recover functionality in the affected areas. In a desperate bid to save the day, Zhang Yazi shared with her husband the oral teaching of the practice. Only a few months have passed, but now he has recovered to the point of being able to walk without crutches! These kinds of examples are extremely numerous. I still do feel that we must practice what we preach. Actual practice is the key, so you mustn't worry about finding definitive proof of its effectiveness a priori. When it comes to health, prevention wins over curing. So, whatever you do, start early, don't leave it to the last minute. Sometimes regret comes too late to save the day."

This is what *sifu* said back then regarding the "Eight Pieces of Brocade." However, owing to the fact that this practice has been passed down lineages for nearly 1,000 years, as one would expect, small additions and omissions have led to slight variations between the techniques of different schools. But this is unimportant; what matters is to be clear about, and master, the key points in every step of the practice. At the time of our studying, we would begin from a standing position, as usual, with feet placed shoulder-width apart. Starting from the *niwangong*[3] acupoint on the crown of

---

3   泥丸宫: The "clay ball palace" acupoint, or GV-20.

the head, we consciously relax the body all the way down to the *yongquan*:[4] every cell, hair follicle, organ, channel, acupoint, bone, and area of skin should relax. Simply put, we should do our utmost to completely relax every area of the body our attention comes to, while regulating the breath until it's comfortable. When doing this practice, gently curl the tongue up to the palate toward the throat while inhaling, then let it rest downward behind the bottom teeth while exhaling. The body and mind are joyful and the face bears a slight smile. When performing the sitting form of the exercises, the relaxation method is largely the same; however, it's best to maintain the legs in lotus position if possible. When my venerable teacher transmitted the "Eight Brocades," there was a handwritten manuscript that he said had been handed down to him from a Daoist priest of the Qing Dynasty. In essence, it was an eight-sentence oral instruction text that employed rhyming verse to aid memorization of the eight key points of the practice. However, according to my knowledge based on the versions of the practice I have seen, some are slower, some are faster, and some have actions added which I had never seen before. Though many are the slight variations, the foundations are indeed all based on the rhyming verse composed of the eight oral instructions.

That year, my teacher also gave me guided instruction regarding the methods in the *Tendon Transformation Classic*. When he transmitted this to me, he added that in fact its predecessor was likely the "Eight Pieces of Brocade." There actually aren't too many aspects we need to pay particular attention to; generally speaking, if the practice can be combined with meditation, the resulting benefits will obviously be even better. Do not do these exercises when feeling very hungry, or when feeling full after eating. Before beginning, you can drink a cup of warm water to better allow the impurities in the body to be flushed out by the practice itself. Starting out, first relax completely until the *laogong* acupoints on both

---

4   湧泉: The "bubbling well" acupoint, or KI-1.

palms feel slightly swollen and warm. During the actual practice, it's best to perform every movement comfortably and slowly.

For example, the first style is called "Two Hands Holding Up the Sky, Aligning the Triple Burner." First adopt the posture previously described, standing with feet shoulder-width apart—it's OK to step out first with either foot. Move the arms forward and interlace the fingers, then lift the hands slowly upward; when they reach the height of the chin, turn them so the palms face the sky, then continue to lift the hands into the space above the head, straightening the arms upward. Both arms should stretch vertically, behind the ears. Following this, the hands separate, the arms moving slowly downward to both sides so that the palms face downward as you slowly return to the beginning stance.

After this, practice the second style, known as "Drawing the Bow Left and Right, Like a Condor." The beginning stance is the same: standing with feet shoulder-width apart, adjust the breathing to become comfortable and even. Clench both hands into fists, at the sides of the body, then step one leg out so that the stance is wider than the shoulders, similar to the crouching posture in horse stance posting. The fists, resting beside the hips, are now brought up in front of the chest, crossing the arms. Relax and unclench the fists, turn the head to the left while the right arm comes up to about shoulder-height, like that of an archer pulling the bow. The right hand sits below the ear, as the left arm rises and extends outward to the left, the *hukou* acupoint (between forefinger and thumb) facing upward. Both eyes glare widely into the distance, looking past space above the *hukou*. After this, once again cross the arms in front of the chest, then stretch the right arm to the right side, as if holding the bow. Repeat the left–right sequence 7 times, then return to the beginning stance.

The following oral instruction is the "Single Arm Stretches to Rejuvenate Spleen and Stomach." The action begins as before, with feet shoulder-width apart: inhale and bring the hands up past the *dantian*, fingers slightly overlapped, palms facing up. As you exhale, rotate one hand completely, and as the palm faces up again, push it up, straightening the arm; at the same time rotate the other hand and push downward, palm facing the ground. The hands then return to the original position when the fingers were crossed in front of the *dantian* area, then the movement repeats with hands switching. Repeat the sequence in this fashion, 7 times.

After completing this exercise, move on to the fourth style, the "Seven Jolts to Eliminate All Illness." The preparatory stance is the same as before: standing with feet shoulder-width apart, regulate the breath 3 times. Then bring the legs together, heels touching, and hands resting by the sides of the legs by the seams of the pants. Inhale and lift the heels off the ground, raise the hands, palms up, to the *tanzhong* at the center of the chest, then begin exhaling and flip the palms to face downward, and swiftly bring the heels back to the ground as the hands return to their original positions beside the thighs. In this way repeat the sequence 7 times.

The fifth style is "Withdraw the Fists and Glare to Increase Vigor." Once again, begin standing with feet shoulder-width apart and regulate the breath 3 times. Then step out to widen your stance, as wide as you would for horse stance posting, clenching your fists on either side of the hips, palms facing upward. After breathing in, begin to move the right fist forward while breathing out, turning the hand so that the palm faces forward. With the *laogong* acupoint thus facing forward, use force to push as if pushing a person. Then rotate the hand 180°, fingers downward, and clench it into a fist again as you inhale and draw the hand back to the hip, exhaling as it reaches the hip. Then do the same with the left arm: inhale first, stretch it out as you exhale, as described above, palm forward as if pushing. Rotate the hand 180° and inhale when bringing the fist back, exhaling just before it reaches the left hip. Repeat the exercise so that each arm performs the movement 7 times. When extending the arm, open up the palm and glare. The practice must be done in full to elicit results. After completing the cycle, return to the original stance. Make sure to combine each practice with appropriate beginning and concluding exercises.

Number six is "Looking Back at Your Illnesses."[5] First, stand comfortably and adjust the breathing 3 times. Then place both hands on the hips, inhale and turn the head toward the right shoulder—do your best to keep the eyes fixed on the right heel. Exhale and return the head back to the forward-facing position, resuming the original stance. Then inhale again and slowly turn the head toward the left shoulder, trying to use your eyes to go look for the left heel. Then exhale as you return the head back to the front, resuming the beginning stance.

Number seven is "Shake the Head and Wag the Tail to Get Rid of Heart Fire." Once again, adjust the breath 3 times while standing, then step out to widen your stance as if you were posting in horse stance. Now place both palms on the knees and prepare to turn the upper body. Inhale, then exhale while slowly moving the right shoulder all the way to the point of touching the left knee. Inhale again and lift the upper body while simultaneously exhaling. Then move the body to the right, and once the upper body and head complete a 360° rotation, return to the original stance. Then inhale again, and as you exhale slowly move the left shoulder to go and touch the right knee. As with the previous movement, make sure the hips, groin, and buttocks move in unison with the upper body as it rotates. In this way, turn to the left and right 7 times each, then resume the original stance.

The final style of the "Eight Brocades" is called "Grabbing the Feet with Two Hands to Strengthen the Lower Back." Stand with feet shoulder-width apart, adjust the breath naturally three times, then cross the hands and relaxedly put them in between the legs, by the *dantian*. Inhale and slowly lift the hands with palms up, until the arms are straight; as the palms turn to face upward, exhale. Then inhale, separate the hands and bow the body forward and down-ward, exhaling slowly until the hands reach the tips of the toes.

---

5   五勞七傷往後瞧 (*wu lao qi shang*): The five in the original name refers to the five viscera: heart, liver, spleen, lungs, and kidneys. The seven refers to the adverse physical effects from overeating (linked to the spleen), anger (liver), moisture (kidney), cold (lung), worry (heart), wind and rain (outer appearance), and fear (mind).

Make sure the legs stay straight, without bend. Then inhale again and return to the original standing posture, and place one hand on top of the other in the center while exhaling. On the next inhalation, repeat the previous movement cycle, a total of seven times, then return to the beginning stance.

CHAPTER 26

CULTIVATING THE MIND TO RETURN TO THE ORIGINAL NATURE—LONGEVITY IS LEVEL WITH THE HEAVENS

There are actually a number of styles of *daoyin* within the schools of Daoism that have been preserved and passed on to this day. These practices of preserving and cultivating health were by no means the monopoly of immortals, but taken up by many prominent figures within the Hundred Schools of Thought.[1] Standing out amongst them was the eminent troublemaker of the Spring and Autumn and Warring States periods, Zhuangzi. He was later given the honorific title within the Daoist schools of "Immortal of the Southern Flower," and left behind at least 100,000 written words for the ages. His disillusionment with the pursuit of status and fortune can be seen throughout his written works, carried by the philosophy of "non-action" and being "at ease." He avoided association with the nobles and officials of his time, and was unconcerned with any criticism his lifestyle and ideas invited. In some circles he had the reputation of shocking and ruffling feathers whenever he opened his mouth; in others he was all the more respected for it. It was those people who believed him to be the veritable embodiment of an immortal, freely coming and going at ease. Zhuangzi didn't pay attention to either camp. He enjoyed passing his days in freedom as he pleased.

The philosophy within Zhuangzi's works is nearly identical

---

1 諸子百家 (*zhu zi bai jia*): Philosophies and schools from the Spring and Autumn period and the Warring States periods of ancient China, 6th century to 221 BCE.

to Laozi's,[2] and the common reverence for both figures within Daoism explains why they are often mentioned in tandem. They both wrote from the central tenet of "following the way of Nature," although Zhuangzi in particular spoke from his experience of the dark, ugly side of politics and human nature. It was because of this that he lived most of his life in revulsion of, and isolation from, the government, believing that all under the state were mere puppets of the emperor. After all, the phrase "being close to the sovereign can be as perilous as lying with a tiger" wouldn't have come about had the emperor not exercised a certain command over the life and death of his subjects. As for Zhuangzi, why not choose a life outside the confines of civilization, a life unbound and unconstrained, a life unhurried and at ease? The spirit of Zhuangzi's thought is that a person should not just wander aimlessly throughout the lands under the sky, but should find a way to thoroughly give expression to their inner world. He lays out some of these ideas central to Daoism in one of his more important essays, *Free and Easy Wandering*.

In another essay, *Ingrained Ideas*, Zhuangzi actually goes into a passage on health cultivation:

Blowing and breathing out through the mouth; inhaling and taking in new, pure air; expelling out all that is dirty, turbulent and unsettled within the heart; stretching and lengthening the body like a black bear [coming out of hibernation], twisting and fluttering like a bird unfurling its wings—those who understand these movements of *daoyin* are far-sighted adepts in nourishing the body and mind, and lengthening the span of their life. They are fond of Peng Zu's long years, in single-minded pursuit of the tortoise's vitality.

Hua Tuo, a famous doctor who lived during the Three Kingdoms period, is the one to concretely put down the "Five Animals" practice for later generations, as a way to bring life to the muscles

---

2 老子 (Laozi): Legendary ancient Chinese philosopher and writer, reputed author of the *Dao De Jing* (the main text of Daoism). The founder of philosophical Daoism, he is revered as a deity in religious Daoism and traditional Chinese religions.

and bones and regulate the breath. Again, the ultimate purpose of this was nourishing and lengthening one's health and life. These movements, however, bring something more like temporary relief rather than treatment of the root causes; the larger aim of Daoism outside of longevity, after all, is the cultivation and correction of the *mind* and a "return to Truth."

Toward this pursuit, no practice is higher than that of "fetal breathing"—a form whereby, in the end, breathing through the nose completely stops. The breath instead reverts to the way we breathed before we were born, in our mother's womb. To achieve this level of breathing requires progression through meditation and exercises with inhalation and exhalation. What begins as somewhat of an artifice ends when you can no longer distinguish whether the breath is there or not. All thought is extinguished, the channels and flow of *qi* stops, and nothing comes in or goes out. One becomes one with Heaven and Earth.

CHAPTER 27

The Change of Miraculous Powers, Crossing Over Eras and Benefiting Life

Rare are those who experience the blossoming of their supernatural abilities after training in Daoist meditation, though this seemed to be more prevalent in China's past. Fei Zhangfang[1] was one such extraordinary individual. A mere officer of a local market, one day Fei had it in his mind to seek out the owner of a medicine shop there. The old herb seller had secretly trained in the arts of the immortals, and Fei had once caught him at the end of the market day jumping into the very gourd that he had used to store and sell his herbs! Fei's curiosity had brewed until he could no longer contain it. He prepared some meat and liquor and waited for his chance to treat the old shop owner to food and drink. Little did he know that not only would the old man accept, but that when Fei paid his visit, the herbalist would pay him back by sucking him right along into his gourd. The world inside the gourd was of an otherworldly beauty—like nothing to be found on Earth. Fei, enchanted, lost all thought of home. After enjoying an evening of splendor within the world of the gourd, the two men returned to the world.

The herbalist told Fei not to speak a word of their journey to anyone. Later, he opened up and revealed who he truly was. The old man, it turns out, had fallen from heaven; he had been amongst the immortals until breaking the laws, and had been sent down to

---

1 費長房: Daoist practitioner and legendary magician from the Eastern Han Dynasty (25–220), known for his supernatural powers.

Earth on probation. His penalty time here, he said, was drawing to a close.

"You and I have a connection," the old man said to Fei. "Come with me to the basement where I store liquor from my private collection. Let's have a drink and say farewell." After asking for directions to the cellar, Fei first sent a man to fetch the liquor. The man returned saying he was unable to move the vessel from its shelf, so Fei went himself with ten others to wrestle the liquor jug from its place, but it wouldn't budge an inch. When the herbalist found out, he chuckled and said, "I'll get it myself, then." When he arrived with the movers in tow, they all watched as, with a single finger, he directed the floating vessel right off the shelf and up the stairs. From appearances, the little jug was only large enough to hold a drink or two, but strangely enough the entire company celebrated through the night as they filled cup after cup from the bottomless jug.

Fei Zhangfang's run-in with the herbalist had actually stirred up a yearning, long suppressed, to learn the ways of the immortals. Since he was a child, his family had prevented him from doing so, and Fei's desire went unfulfilled until chancing upon the old herbalist and the gourd. He told the old man of his long-buried wish, and the old man said, "It shouldn't be that hard!" He went outside, snapped off a stalk of bamboo, and came back to measure Fei's height. "When you go home tonight, hang this bamboo stalk inside your bedroom," the herbalist said.

Whatever the bamboo stick's power, the entire family thought that Fei had passed away in his room that night. They mourned, and arranged for his funeral. Fei came to his own funeral procession with his casket to reveal himself, only to realize that there wasn't a single person in the procession who could see him. He was, for all intents and purposes, gone. Although his "passing" was tragic to those around him, Fei followed the course of this fortuitous occasion and vanished to learn the Dao with the old herbalist.

During his time studying with the "Old Immortal from the Gourd," Fei witnessed many incredible and unbelievable things.

When his training was finished and it was time to part, the old immortal handed him the bamboo stick once more. "From now on, this bamboo stick will become your horse. Wherever you wish to travel, it will take you to your destination," he said. He also handed Fei a talisman he had painted himself. "With this, you can command any spirit that walks upon the earth," he said.

Fei took the gifts and "rode" off, arriving instantly at the doorsteps of his family home. "It must be only a few days since I left," he thought.

When he listened around town and put the pieces together, he realized that more than ten years had passed! As the story goes, he threw his bamboo staff into the town lake and was shocked to watch it transform into a dragon. Upon returning home, he faced his entire family's disbelief. "If you don't believe me, let us go and dig up my grave to find out the truth," Fei said. When they opened up the casket, indeed the only thing left inside was a single stick of bamboo. Needless to say, the family changed their minds.

Fei Zhangfang also had the unique talent of being able to cure people wherever he went, using skills learned from his Daoist training. If the illness was spirit-induced, Fei would fix the person right up with a simple whack from his whip. Any spirits within range of his power would fall under his command if he so chose. On those occasions, he could be seen looking slightly deranged, all in a huff and muttering to himself. When asked what the problem was, he would reply, saying things like "It's nothing, I'm just giving my piece of mind to those law-breaking spirits." These are the stories I heard in abundance in my youth. As for Fei Zhangfang, it was said that he met his end at the hands of the spirits after the talisman given to him by the old herbalist went missing.

There is an endless cast of Daoist immortals from history, each with their own uncanny abilities. Some could move objects over huge distances; some could disappear, remaining practically invisible while standing right in front of you; some could transform into whatever form they desired, becoming man or woman at will; some could shapeshift animals into human form; some could stay underwater indefinitely, or stand consumed by fire for three days and nights without a single burn; some could chop their bodies into pieces; some could see things from thousands of miles away.

A Daoist priest once told me a story over dinner about a practitioner of the Dragon Gate Sect called Priest Li. Li, a stocky, sturdy, and uneducated fellow, had once been a long-term hired hand on a wealthy estate. Later on, he was swept up by fortune and placed at the feet of a master of the Longmen School, with whom he began to travel and train in the Dao. When he descended from the mountains years later, Li was a different man, reminiscent of Chan master Daoji. Disheveled, vagrant, and often singing wildly in words no one understood, Priest Li would just whimsically appear on the doorsteps of people's homes. Beating his hand drum and singing, he said on one occasion that he was helping someone in the household pass on, that the old man was going to a good place. Less than two days later, the old man passed away. Another time, he walked straight into a residence, without permission or request, and began yelling and hitting the man of the house. When he was done, he demanded money for his "medical services." That same family had just two days earlier emptied their pockets to bring in the area's best doctor to treat the father for imbalances of wind in the body, to no effect. Little did they expect that the minute the raving, violent Li stepped out of the house, the father got up and started walking as if he had never been sick.

Another time, Li charged straight for the head of the largest estate in the county, looking furious and demanding an audience while he struggled against the estate's guards. The whole lot of them could not so much as deter Li an inch, and like a bull he barged through and roared his request. As soon as the owner came out, Li pounced and slapped him twice on the face. He hammered away at the man, hollering curses and things no one could really make out. In fact, no one could make out what had even incurred the mad Daoist's wrath in the first place. Days later, the same owner was out surveying his lands, picking his way along a ravine. The path gave out from under him, and he slipped right off the edge, plummeting into the depths. It surely would have been the end of his life, but he swore he felt someone pull him by the sleeve, yanking him toward a thick, outlying tree branch jutting out over the ravine. Snagged on the branch, he hung there thrashing and yelling, scared senseless but unhurt, life still clinging to him.

The priest telling me the story wasn't able to say just how many lives this Priest Li had saved, but there Li was, warning people of impending disaster between a cackle and a curse, yet always there to snatch them away from danger when it struck.

It was actually in the depths of winter that he and Priest Li had first met, the priest said. They were traveling in a group to a mountain temple. Everyone was bundled up in wool coats and thick robes save Li, showing not the slightest awareness of the cold in his short-sleeved shirt. Among the others was the householder Yi Huang. When they were coming back down the mountain, Yi Huang swore he could feel an inexplicable warmth radiating off Li's body. It was so sweltering that Yi Huang broke out in a sweat just sitting next to him. This was enough to demonstrate the extraordinary level of Priest Li's inner cultivation. The only reason he was fortunate enough to meet Li, the priest continued, was on the chance request of one of Li's disciples, the abbot of a temple, to make that very visit.

Li himself was a man of few words. He wouldn't always answer when spoken to, but there was always a brightness in his eyes that made it hard to look at him directly. That day at the temple, as Li was politely escorting the group out and they prepared to depart, the visiting priest could not help but note that, in his inspection of Li's skin he found no signs of aging. With such pure skin and no visible wrinkles, it was hard to even make a guess about his age. Needless to say, it would have been impolite to ask. The abbot did reveal a little in their conversation as they made their way back, saying that Li rarely spoke, and spent almost all of his time in meditation. There was even one night, when the abbot paid a visit to Li's quarters to make a request, that he noticed a dim light glowing out from one the cracks of the screen doors. He peered through and saw the Daoist adept sitting, looking like a bright, clear beacon shrouded in what seemed to be a mist. Not knowing what to make of the light, the abbot decided to find another time to make his request and left quietly.

And yet, despite the multitude of wondrous accounts we have of the immortals, of their displays of power, in the end they are merely a display, and not the ultimate essence. The ultimate reality of the so-called "True Man" of the immortal is *chuhua*, *ruhua*—the immortal state words cannot possibly depict. It is a state that cannot be measured, quantified, or explained by modern science. It is a state beyond any thoughts or ideas imaginable in our universe. It is not simply the means to capture longevity; it goes totally beyond it. Whether or not a seeker can attain such a state depends on whether they can reach the point where "the soul dies, yet doesn't depart." The principle and practice of meditation never deviates from this: externally, practice and train in the form; internally, transform and align with the Truth. This process, assisted by the various Daoist exercises (in breathing and physical forms), eventually builds in the practitioner the extension of his or her life. Throughout this transformation, there is nothing more difficult than keeping the six roots—the five senses and one's thoughts—from drifting outward, without being affected by worldly pursuits and desires. It requires no small effort to successfully and completely let go of these. It is an undeniable challenge to see through the great worldly concerns: one's reputation, success, and fortune; desire for food, sleep, and sex; excessive self-preservation in matters of life and death; or whether one passes the life of a king or a beggar.

CHAPTER 28

Neither Grasping nor Guarding, a Myriad Originations Are Let Go Of

Although meditation belongs to the path of internal alchemy, the ultimate can't merely be contained within the oft-seen longevity methods. Whether the practitioner attains, through the dual cultivation of body and mind, a state wherein he or she is replete both physically and spiritually, where the Dao and phenomena are within one's grasp, where one melds seamlessly with phenomena, this practitioner is still far from the ultimate method. An immortal of lore once said: "The light behind the peak seems like an illusion; one may fly above the clouds, yet not be an immortal." This shows us that although we may have overcome the limitations of an ordinary person to become a saint, the key remains cultivating one's mind. Only this is the ultimate.

In the late 1970s, I had a chance to meet a Daoist priest who came to Taiwan from mainland China. He was already in his eighth or ninth decade and had once served as the general manager of a public service department. From early on, he had a deep connection with Daoism, and his life's practice was centered on upholding some of the key points from the *Yellow Court Classic*. At that time, there were very few people in Taiwan who were knowledgeable about this text. On one occasion, I fortuitously came to know that the priest was deeply versed in the esoteric instructions within the Classic, including its "Internal View" and "External View" sections. Overjoyed at this unexpected discovery, I decided to visit him.

This venerable Daoist elder spilled out his several decades of experience and understanding without withholding a single drop, leaving me filled with the joy of an unexpected harvest. The gist of what he shared was that in one's meditation, one should not obsess over techniques of guarding the acupoints, for these are all methods within "form," and thus removed from the superior aspects of Daoism. When regulating the breath in meditation, if you have not yet reached the stage where breath seems internal yet isn't, seems external yet isn't, where there is only one, unimpeded breath that seems to breathe with Heaven and Earth, slightly dazed and silent like you are residing in primal chaos…you have, in fact, not reached even the beginning stage of meditation. From the elementary perspective of "utmost emptiness and silence," the first step is to build a foundation and cultivate warmth through meditation. Then, by circulating the chariot, one's governing and conception channels are freed of obstacles, until one enters the state of "fetal breathing," where the mind and breath experience not the slightest leakage. By preserving and protecting this life-force, the *qi* will gradually flow smooth and unimpeded throughout all channels, and the mind will become illumined. If one can then maintain this state, the pill of immortality can be obtained.

I learned so very much from this meeting. This Daoist elder also expounded less elevated concepts to a fellow practitioner, saying that when you are circulating the chariot, you must put your attention on the *dantian* and not let your mind or spirit wander. The tip of the tongue is placed on the palate, just behind the teeth, and once the mouth fills with saliva it stirs it around; you can then swallow this sweet, ambrosia-like saliva, and it will help regulate your heart fire. For this, you need the mind and breath to be united, the latter extremely fine and soft, with the upper and lower jaw set firmly, the six orifices tightly sealed, and vigilant attention. The elder explained that there is a reason behind this: when circulating the chariot, if the top is not sealed, the fire *qi* cannot amalgamate, and if this fire *qi* is insufficient, you cannot concoct the pill. The reasoning for the descending *qi* is the same. Both the ascending and descending *qi* must be sealed for there to be a chance of focusing the spirit and concocting the pill. He repeatedly and kindly admonished us to be extremely vigilant during this crucial segment of one's practice, lest there be true danger to our health.

In addition, the Daoist said that his predecessors during the Qing Dynasty had passed down the practice of the "Five Animals"—the five being the tiger, deer, bear, monkey, and bird. External martial artists then appropriated the methods and renamed them, but they essentially used these to cultivate their essence, *qi*, strength, bones, and spirit. The venerable elder also demonstrated the movements, and it was a feast for the eyes.

This elder Daoist had spent a very long time in meditation since his youth, so he gave some more pertinent suggestions: "The most important thing in meditation is not to keep store of delusional thoughts, because this induces 'fire,' and if it becomes a habit it can easily cause tinnitus and rising fire, i.e., a lack of *yin* in the body. If this internal heat scuttles its way into other channels, the skin can easily break into rashes or red patches. If the heat rises into the viscera, it will turn the spirit and soul topsy-turvy and this will cause restless sleep filled with unsettling dreams. During meditation, don't think of gain and fame, nor get stuck on any thought or emotion, nor get alarmed; rather, focus simply on the subtlety and depth of your breath. Whatever state of mind or situation comes up, remain poised in equanimity, whether it is good or bad, just don't pay it any heed." At this time, the elder priest also taught us how to pluck the small and big medicine, and how to use external breathing, how to regulate the rise and fall, coming and going of the internal breath without causing rising fire. He particularly emphasized that one must reach the stage of "plucking without plucking" to achieve the best physical results. Very patiently, he explained when we should stop and when we should apply more effort, how we should regulate the breath when the *yang qi* is in excess so as to prevent the rise of fire *qi*, how to gradually regulate the breath, how to gradually use the rise of *yin* after the noontime in order to reduce fire.

The Daoist priest told us that young practitioners like us need to not look upon meditation as something too serious, something to be scared of. Really, all you need is to maintain an equal, smooth, natural breath, and the spirit will gradually coalesce so that your mind is left with a permeating feeling of ease, neither fast nor slow, neither neglecting states nor following them—mind and *qi* united, not controlled by phenomena internal or external, until you reach the purity and harmony of Heaven and Earth. He also told us that if those with a sturdy foundation can contain their mind and spirit, they can naturally increase their store of true *qi*; however, this only applies when at the beginning of the harmonization of the fire and water elements there's an impetus of *yang qi*. The practice method employed must be the correct one, and if the method is correct, then one can succeed in using essence to replenish one's cognitive capabilities. In regard to the practice throughout daily life, after you get up from the meditation cushion, you must understand how to collect the mind and spirit and minimize distracted thoughts. Whatever activity you engage in, don't let the mind and spirit scatter out and about, and you will accumulate *qi*. Don't pay attention to any of the thoughts that come up in your mind. Even were you to feel the onset of psychic powers, pay it no heed; do not rejoice or get angry. You must accustom yourself to the unusual, so that these experiences have no hold on you. Meld humbly and seamlessly within the clamor of the world, with a mind empty and free of any constraints. Real meditation is indeed such, occurring in the midst of the loud, confused cacophony of the city, where your mind doesn't give rise to the slightest differentiation, least of all to any thoughts of anger and hatred.

As soon as an individual's thoughts become excessive and their temper flares, this will transform into harmful fire. The Daoist elder said he had spent decades of his life working on these very things: he believed that to be able to still and pacify the mind, to deal with things as they come and let them go without a trace once dealt with, allows our genuine true mind to come to the surface, and pure *yang qi* to arise. By conserving essence, *qi*, and spirit in this manner over a long time, one can attain great health and longevity.

This was truly a marvelous spiritual connection on the path of the Dao! In these encounters, perhaps owing to his realization that his remaining days were scant, the Daoist elder revealed to us young aspiring practitioners not only all of the aforementioned advice, but also many stories of his own meetings and spiritual connections with virtuous, accomplished masters and immortals of the past. During that period, we visited him perhaps four or five times, our meetings ranging from a couple hours long to most of the day, and with the utmost patience he answered each and every one of the questions we brought to him. This kind of largesse and self-restraint was truly a worthy inspiration for us and the following generations.

CHAPTER 29

THE GREAT POOL OF DESIRE—TABOOS OF DAOIST CULTIVATORS

There is an ancient poem, "A Lifetime Does Not Reach a Hundred Years," that goes as follows:

> *A lifetime does not reach a hundred years*
> *Yet it ever contains the sorrow of a thousand years*
> *When days be short, and bitter nights long*
> *Why not grasp one's lamp and roam about?*
> *Happiness is found at present without delay*
> *How could one wait for it to come here?*
> *The fool cherishes his wealth,*
> *Yet in later years is laughed at*
> *Master Wang became a stately immortal,*
> *Such an achievement would be much to hope for*

This poem describes the plight of the average person: although they know that their worldly life is impermanent, they cannot overcome the allure of material things. They act as if fame and fortune were treasures that will last forever. Indeed, our lives are like a drop of dew on a blade of grass. And though most people realize how precious and fleeting their existence is, they are unable to break the bind that pretty things have on their way of living. Though they witness that good and bad things all fade away, and they know that human life is fleeting, they cannot resist superficial pleasures. Many people know the importance of practicing internal cultivation and doing good deeds to accumulate virtue, but they lack resolve to give up the things that make them stumble. Thus, they often stray unintentionally, stirring up bad karma that will trouble them for 1,000 years hence. The greatest challenge for Daoist practitioners is to recognize impermanence and the power of karma. These are fixed laws of reality—they cannot be altered. People know perfectly well that their possessions will all end up on a trash heap, yet they continue to struggle with attachment rather than gracefully let things go. Visiting graveyards, people understand that the spirits beneath don't think of returning to some fixed place. As they hurry away from the cemetery, perhaps they hear the desolate howl of the wind rushing through nearby cypress and pine trees. In such moments, people feel disconsolate; they cannot ignore the reality of impermanence. But as soon as they turn from such a place, they forget these feelings; they let the tide of their old impulses and desires overtake them.

Common people are familiar with the sacred accounts of Daoist immortals and their sublime ascensions. But who knows of the untold many who pursued immortality and instead met untimely deaths? Few among us have a destiny like that of the son of Zhou Ling Wang, Wang Qiao. He rode a crane through the skies toward the Western Paradise, and along the way met a Daoist immortal who was a master alchemist. The alchemist taught the prince techniques for achieving longevity. For decades thereafter, the prince's family members and the common folk all thought he had died. In fact, he had passed through the clouds on the back of that white crane, and transcended into immortality. It was altogether miraculous.

Over the course of my time at *sifu*'s residence, studying meditation and the Daoist arts, I was fortunate to observe numerous changes in the secular world. At that time, my fellow Daoist practitioners comprised three or four groups. Some meditation groups had many people and some had relatively few, but in most classes there were over 100 attendees. Because of *sifu*'s compassion, I often stayed on as the classes changed, and continued to study. I came away from each session with new insights. In this way, I not only learned about meditation and received oral tips, but I also had the opportunity to be near *sifu* and attend to him. The latter experience was the most instructive of all. From the disciples that came and went, I observed much about the vicissitudes of bureaucracy and status. Among *sifu's* students were former landlords who had lost everything in a single night. Just like that, they went from presiding over vast estates to living in destitution.

One of the people I got to know was the heir of an extremely wealthy Tainan family. A fellow Daoist in our order introduced the man to *sifu*, and thereafter he began to study meditation with us. He drove up from Tainan every week to join the courses on Daoist cultivation. This Mr. Wu was around 40 when he joined our practice. He was a dignified-looking man, bespectacled, and of medium build. He had earned a master's degree abroad and held an important position in his family's enterprise. In every regard, Mr. Wu's manner indicated that he was a modest, disciplined gentleman. However, after spending more time around him, I realized that he had many of the faults typical to men. He was married, but had long been keeping a mistress, and indulged in all sorts of bad habits. He entertained year round and lived wantonly as a socialite, drinking and smoking constantly. In the end, he passed away prematurely. Mr. Wu was not yet 50 when he died.

Day to day in meditation, he had exuded such integrity and prudence. He showed no arrogance nor impatience in his studies, and he always acted with propriety. In these moments, an observer would find it difficult to believe that he was a businessman who acted without loyalty to his wife and children. *Sifu*, in his wisdom, likely had a more complete understanding of Mr. Wu from the beginning. More than once, I overheard *sifu* courteously instruct him that he must take strict care not to indulge in lust for women. Moreover, *sifu* clearly explained to Mr. Wu that conserving essence through abstinence and mitigating all desires were critical disciplines in cultivating the Dao and progressing in meditation. But perhaps the simple truth is that people's cravings are sometimes too vast; satisfying them is like trying to level a ravine. This Wu fellow surely knew that *sifu*'s teachings, while bitter to swallow, were good for him. Nevertheless, no sooner would he cross back into the outer world that any semblance of self-control would vanish. Like a housefly on rotting meat, he was loath to tear himself away from temptations. We were about 20 years apart in age. I remember how he often spoke to me back then, helpless and embarrassed: "Good grief, man, these troubles of mine would probably be tough for you to understand. We're from different worlds. Maybe this will make sense to you one day, but for now there's no way I can tell you about what's going on."

Mr. Wu had mentioned how, by day, he was always pressed to rush around, tending to various business matters and maintaining the company's bottom line; and by night he was obliged to entertain clients. Almost every evening he went out drinking with various contacts, just to secure business deals. He once accidentally revealed that this lifestyle was tremendously distressing to him, but most of the time when the matter came up he just brushed it off, saying, "It's not so bad; it's all fine!" Every day, he practiced the foundational meditation methods *sifu* had taught him, including "fetal breathing" and posting—otherwise I imagine he may have died even younger.

The secular world is full of unfortunate binds, and you cannot have your cake and eat it too. This is especially true for people in bureaucratic positions or businessmen. I suppose it's like the line in Huang Zunxian's poem "Sighs of the Woman Next Door": "From afar drift sounds of senior officials in the great halls; But for all the carousing, satisfaction has yet to arrive." Or as He Jingming said: "Who can claim that wealth and fame are the way to blessedness? For the proud and extravagant, disaster is always near." Sometimes our environment shapes us in ways we can't control. It may be that only the people who experience such pressures first-hand actually learn this lesson. The culture of debauchery that surrounded Mr. Wu pushed him to entertain Japanese clients and other foreign businessmen. In those days, the Beitou hot spring district was the most popular destination for people visiting from abroad. Mr. Wu often went there with his guests, and he was always expected to bring along girls to sing and carouse with them. Over the course of these outings, he fell head over heels for a certain escort's flashy attire and lithe figure. He thought nothing of the difference between their ages, and just like that, his days of contentment and fidelity as a married man were over.

Matters of sex have always been a stumbling block to seekers of the Dao. Those who are serious about attaining longevity must avoid these entanglements, as one would a wild tiger or wolf. Even though Mr. Wu knew that such tigers and wolves roamed the proverbial mountain, he veered toward the mountain path and the inevitable consequences that awaited him there. Indeed, his days were numbered. Both his body and mind were worn out, and his kidney water was totally depleted. The result was the onset of all kinds of illnesses and, eventually, he couldn't hold onto life any longer. His story demonstrates that those who cultivate the Daoist arts and seek to refine their *qi* must maintain a sound body and mind. In these practices, nothing is more important than outer and inner tranquility, purity, and self-control. Over the many years I've been involved with meditation and the broad community of practitioners, I have met countless people with destinies like Mr. Wu's.

In the earlier days when Mr. Wu was still around, he told me in private that he had met an old Daoist from the Southern School who studied Daoist "bedroom arts." I had previously warned him about wayward Daoist sects and their unorthodox methods, explaining that, if possible, he should not get involved with them. He may well have thought it all through or had some real needs driving his interest; I wouldn't have considered this possibility back then. I had heard about the teachings of such sects from numerous practitioners of older generations. In the beginning, they thought the methods were reliable and the results sound, but of course the instructors were not true Daoist saints in the traditional sense. Though they practiced internal cultivation, they failed to achieve immortality. If the teachings in these areas are not correct, and a practitioner proceeds with the slightest slip in caution, they will easily go overboard. They may become possessed or otherwise become distracted by dangerous phenomena or trivialities from their meditations. I had spoken about these matters before with an elder Daoist saint by the name of Wu Liu, who came to Taiwan from Guangdong. In his youth in mainland China, he had practiced these niche Daoist methods. When I visited him, the fates aligned that he would discuss his views on these matters with me. He explained that originally these practices were not evil; rather, a few sectarian leaders, claiming affiliation with the Southern School, had misused them to attract new followers. The real purpose of the original Daoist sexual practices was not to indulge lust; rather, they were developed to help mitigate the harms of sex and to facilitate conservation of essence. That is to say, the techniques were meant to help practitioners protect their vitality. There are numerous methods in this category. If transmitted from an upright teacher, practitioners may use them to recover essence, boost *qi*, and, through *qi*, support their spirit. Some people can slow the aging process and even regain youthful vigor through the correct use of these methods.

Elder Wu Liu said that he had begun exploring this type of practice out of curiosity when he was a young man. He studied with five or six masters of the sect, and their teachings more or less covered supplementation of deficiencies, mitigation of severe losses or damage, and means of gathering *yin* and boosting *yang*. I was also curious, and asked the veteran practitioner if he had any reliable literature on hand that I might reference to learn more. Wu Liu responded: "It's best to not waste too much time on these teachings. Don't follow the same path I did." It turns out that many of the books associated with this sect are full of incorrect teachings fabricated by people who came after the original practitioners. The authors often claim to be drawing from the wisdom of the Yellow Emperor and Goddess Su Nu and their books—the *Yellow Emperor's Classic of Internal Medicine*, and the *Classic of the White Madame*, respectively—taking advantage of their reputations to popularize sham practices. In a nutshell, almost all of the literature associated with this sect promotes false theories and methods. Without truly enlightened teachers and sufficient transmission of the authentic methods—that is, without masters who can serve as virtuous guides for subsequent generations of practitioners—the result is mortal harm.

Sun Simiao's *Bei Ji Qian Jin Yao Fang,* (*Essential Formulas for Emergencies Worth a Thousand Pieces of Gold*) actually includes an essay on the benefits of the original Daoist sexual practices. However, the text mainly admonishes people who have passed middle age to protect and store up a surplus of essence. It is not at all about single-minded pursuit of sensual gratification. If those who engage with these methods do not exercise self-control, their practice is tantamount to suicide. Caution is essential.

Relevant classical texts employ all sorts of obtuse phrases in their discussions of this subject: "how to calm the furnace," "how to cast the sword," "how to draw water and rekindle fire," "how to use the three yellow ointments," "restoring, moving, and transforming the original *qi*," etc. In fact, these are all euphemisms. Elder Wu Liu, a true master of these techniques, translated the bizarre terms into plain language for me, and the meanings were suddenly clear. This proves that an authentic transmission can be expressed in a few words. But, alas, over the course of history, how many people have exhausted their life-force on account of these arcane practices.

Like so many men, Mr. Wu was always hoping he could satisfy the woman in his life. His entrée into schemes of self-improvement to this end was the ingestion of folk tonics. Later, he was introduced to someone from Taiwan who claimed to be a *qigong* master, and this "master" taught him so-called "essence washing techniques." Mr. Wu spent enormous sums of money in this process and held himself to daily applications of ointment, ingestion of tonic, and all sorts of other things. This menagerie of treatments put him in an unstable frame of mind. He was confused and distracted and eventually began to look sickly as well. His skin yellowed and his body wasted away. In the end, he was poisoned through overuse of the medicines. The master who had been advising him in these matters had admonished him repeatedly not to overdo it, but the warnings had no effect. Perhaps there was nothing to be done all along, and it just happened according to karmic destiny.

CHAPTER 30

DEPART FROM WORRY AND EMOTIONALITY— THE EIGHT HURDLES OF DAOIST PRACTICE

What is it that people long for?
Desire flows toward two extremes,
Ordinary people pine after fame and fortune,
Those of lofty spirit want to be like the saints,
The realm of immortals is a tight-knit club,
Fame and fortune are also decided by the heavens,
Do not crave the life of politics and parties,
And seek not the sacred mountains,
The Western Capital is a swirl of dust
The Eastern Sea, an endless sway of waves…

This poem was written by Bai Juyi. Throughout his life, he immersed himself in Confucianism, Buddhism, and Taoism. He diligently studied Buddhism and Chan but was especially drawn to the way of the Daoist immortals. The profound ease with which they moved through the world inspired awe bordering on fear. Bai Juyi understood that though countless people seek the Dao, only a few reach enlightenment. True immortals are as scarce as rare jewels.

Bai Juyi was not the only one who recognized this idea; throughout history it has been commonly understood. Many people want to merge with the Dao and become immortal, but they can't let go of their fixations on reputation and wealth. Learned, cultured people [have experienced this tension] since ancient times.

From within wealthy society and the halls of power, they looked to the Daoist saints with admiration. [But admiration is insufficient]; seekers must be prepared to fully relinquish their hold on all trappings of the secular world. Single-minded devotion is required to cultivate the Dao. Riches and honor, life and death—[true practitioners] recognize that all such things are as transient as the clouds. The [travails and vanities] of the past are plain to observe, but somehow people can't grasp them. It may depress people to reflect on the impermanence of this world. All human affairs are fleeting. People come and go; this is the way of things. No wonder the literary greats wrote most often of the parting between people:

At dawn, the traveler sings a song of parting
Last night, fine frost just crossed the Yellow River
The cries of the wild geese so sorrowful to hear
Let alone the clouds and mountain a traveler must pass
In the gate of the city, daybreak brings on such chill,
And the pounding sounds of the capital bring on the night
Don't think of Chang'an as a place to seek pleasures
Or precious months and precious years will vainly pass by

The author of this poem, Li Qi, lived during the Tang Dynasty. His environment afforded ample opportunities to meet Daoist alchemists who were skilled in inner cultivation. As a result, he also became well versed in these arts. It is said that well into Li Qi's old age, his skin remained clear and rosy, with no wrinkles to be seen. He had a magnanimous spirit and was prone to grand gestures, always ready to take up the cause of the needy. His network extended far and wide, and he treated his friends with extreme generosity. Li Qi gave away such vast sums of money and property that he didn't have enough for himself to live on.

Eventually, the messiness of human affairs drove him from secular society. He felt that the worldly life didn't hold anything for him any longer, and he began studying the *Yellow Court Classic*. As he considered leaving civilization for the life of a hermit, he shed all vulgarities, and his manner became refined and pure. Much of Li Qi's writing on these themes has been passed down through subsequent generations.

As a young man, he had put great effort into achieving honor and rank, studying hard for the imperial exams. Once he became an official, however, his performance was unremarkable. Near the end of his life, he gave special gravity to matters of affection. He was sensitive by nature, and sorrow overtook him every time he had to bid a friend farewell. The afore-quoted poem demonstrates this tender disposition. Li Qi's friend is merely traveling to the capital city to sit for the imperial exam. Yet even the temporary separation evoked such sorrow in the poet that he penned these melancholy verses.

On the surface, the poem describes an elder's earnest well wishes to a young person [in parting], but the sense of melancholy it captures is broadly resonant. Whether evoked by a thin frost at dawn, or the brays of wild geese as they pass over a lake, or perhaps the chill of a mourner at a graveside on an autumn night, this is the universal ache of separation that reverberates throughout Li Qi's poem.

Du Mu[1] also wrote a poem in this vein:

Much warmth and affection in the end feels cold,
I feel that before I drink, a smile is unable to form.
The candle has a heart, laments even departure,
And bears in our stead till daybreak, the task of shedding tears.

Du Mu is a distinctive figure in the world of Chinese poetry. He was extremely talented with both the pen and sword. It is said that he was an innovative military strategist. However, he was never as fortunate in his official career as his grandfather, Duke Anjian of Qi. Moreover, Du Mu was caught up in the factional strife between

---

1   杜牧 (Du Mu): Tang Dynasty poet (803–852).

Niu Sengru and Li Deyu[2] throughout his life, and the turmoil made him ill at ease. Consequently, he was often in an unquiet state of mind.

As it was, neither Niu nor Li could ever determine the true allegiances of Du Mu, who seemed to just go with the flow of the political tides. In fact, Du Mu never directly stated his position to either of the faction leaders. He was meant to be a man of letters, and he could not contain the particular haughtiness of a born scholar. It was with this nature that he had borne the decades of political conflict, and as a result he had matured into a mournful figure. In his daily life, he could only find emotional release in the world of brothels and sensual entertainment. He also turned to fellow poets, who saw his plight. These friends not only understood him; they also understood the inner life, and their sympathies consoled Du Mu. Thus, friendship held special value for him. Every time a close companion departed, he could not contain his feelings and would pour them into verse. Consider the poem quoted here: though the meeting described is brief, it showcases a profound bond. The verses convey such strength of attachment, the reader can't help but feel the warmth [of connection]. But this warmth is a fleeting joy in the face of separation! Like the candle on the table, glowing from its burning wick, its light brings it nearer to its own end. The fire at its center heralds its impermanence, and the wax tears can only roll down in silence. The candles cry on behalf of the people, accompanying them until daybreak.

The Chinese poetry canon overflows with these descriptions of farewell scenes because people are emotional creatives. Of the

---

2 牛僧孺, 李德裕: Two court officials representing factions in an ongoing contention at the court of the mid- to late Tang dynasty. The Niu Faction (牛黨), named after Niu Sengru, was largely viewed as a faction of officials with humble origins who passed the imperial examinations to get into government. The Li Faction (李黨), named after Li Deyu, was largely viewed as a faction of officials with aristocratic origins.

eight distresses,[3] this, the pain of parting, is the most difficult to overcome in seeking the Dao. But within the Dao, affection and its absence are the same. A great number of poems describe the sad haze of parting. Some of them use beautiful language to foreground the people's heartfelt regard for each other, but the overarching tone of reluctance is clear. And some poets attempt to drum up feelings of strength and encouragement, but they fail to hide their true desolation, and the reader comes away with a melancholy that's hard to shake off. These ideas have appeared in all sorts of formulations: "from time immemorial, how many bonds have existed; how many painful goodbyes exchanged?", "the depths of dejection lie in words of farewell", and "the grief of separation cannot be cut off, cannot be neatly managed"... The theme is ubiquitous across literary genres and songs from throughout history. These expressive works capture the experience of powerful feelings and the adversity that they engender. Between couples and in all the familial relations, any issues that reach the emotional level end up affecting the mindset of everyone in the household. So, of course, such sentiments also present difficulties for the process of internal cultivation. All of the esteemed teachers, elders, and priests I have met with over the years have cautioned me: on the practitioner's journey, the most formidable challenges are the feelings between men and women, and nocturnal emissions. These two hurdles have been the greatest impediment to seekers across eras, and they cannot be ignored.

---

3 八苦 (baku): Birth, old age, sickness, death, separation from loved ones, association with those we dislike, unfulfilled wishes and desires, suffering as inseparable from the nature of the Five Skandhas/Aggregates. These eight distresses refer to the fundamentally unsatisfying, painful nature of mundane life according to Buddhism. In particular, the last one maintains that suffering is inseparable from the very nature of these five aggregates—form, sensations, perceptions, mental activity and consciousness—that play a large part in our own idea of "I," of who and how we are, as mistakenly distinct from the world around us. While the five are ultimately empty of independent existence (as is everything else), humans give rise to all their suffering by clinging to these factors, thus ensuring their continuation of existence in saṃsāra, with its uninterrupted cycle of life–death–rebirth. In Mahāyāna Buddhism, the point of spiritual practice is indeed to break free of the five, break free of saṃsāra (by realizing the emptiness of all things), and go beyond, becoming enlightened for the benefit of all sentient beings.

CHAPTER 31

THE CAREFUL TRANSMISSION OF A WISE MASTER—ON MANAGING MEDITATION-INDUCED ERECTION

I gave you the example of my fellow practitioner Wu, whose main issue revolved around romantic relationships. The truth is that when it comes to desires, and regardless of your gender, if you are unable to understand the issue at hand, clearly thus letting it go, it can become an issue plaguing you throughout your lifetime. This is particularly true for those who have just started to take up meditation. They will likely have the issue of meditation-induced erection during their sitting and find themselves unable to overcome it. I often see some diligent fellow meditators, some of whom even sit several times a day and exert themselves greatly, all running into this issue. Though they might know how to handle it in principle, out of ignorance and lack of meditative stillness most eventually give in.

Beginners in particular find it challenging to resist the temptation [to release the pressure thus induced through ejaculation]. The meditation-induced erection usually occurs when the sun is about to set. This is the time of day when *yin* and *yang* alternate, hence the elements of water and fire meet. Owing to their abundant *yang qi*, youngsters and those in their prime of life are likely to run into this situation. When meditation-induced erection occurs, there are six time periods that practitioners ought to seize in order to move on to the next stage of "replete *qi* whence one can collect the medicine." Since people's capacity and motivation vary, practitioners should understand the principle well and know how to use it to avoid squandering the opportunity. And that is all I can say here. In the past, unless you received the teachings from your own master, caution should be exercised, otherwise you might end up making a futile attempt by following obscure instructions on how to move the *qi* alongside the channel pathways. What Chinese Medicine, or even Western Medicine, offers in terms of the *ren* and *du* channels diagram is somewhat different from the Daoist Inner Alchemy School based on the teachings of senior practitioners I personally heard it from. Over many past years, I have been asked about this several times. The position that past sages and holy men took is that unless a disciple has been observed rigorously for their upright character for several years, as far as I know, a master would not rashly pass the oral tips on. Therefore, I can only hope that fellow practitioners exercise special caution.

Those who wish to attain the foundational level of Daoist Elixir of Youth through meditation should base their practice on the principle that one's mind is interconnected with the kidneys.[1] You need a qualified and experienced teacher to point out how to correctly use alternately gentle or forceful methods in order to rarify essence into *qi* and form the elixir (*dan*). After this stage, however, each school has its own methods. Some emphasize the oral tips of circulating the cosmic orbit to achieve a warm *dantian*. This, however, requires a careful study of the interaction between one's spirit and *qi*. It should never be blindly following methods of ascending and descending the *qi*, some of which are not only unsuitable but downright flawed. It is said that the slightest difference leads to a huge loss. One should definitely be cautious. The initial method one employs should be the correct one. To the best of my knowledge, a dozen fellow practitioners spent over two or three decades [trying], but unfortunately still failed to produce the pill.

---

1   心神不離腎水 (*xin shen bu li shen shui*): According to Chinese Medicine, the mind belongs to the fire element, while the kidneys are a "water" organ system. It is of paramount importance to keep the two in a state of balance, as all psychophysical ailments are caused by imbalances in the elements of the body.

In short, there are so many bizarre instructions out there whose legitimacy is yet to be proved, only practitioners of great merit can encounter authentic ones.

A visiting fellow practitioner from Singapore told me that a Daoist teacher who came to teach in Singapore from Fujian once told him that when meditation-induced erection occurred, simply swish the tongue to produce a generous amount of saliva then swallow it. He consulted me on this method, but I couldn't allow myself to be too frank with him. In my mind, however, I knew it's true that saliva produced as a result of one's meditation is rich in different enzymes, but that's all. Some even teach an incorrect method to "obtain" *qi* and recklessly give instructions on how to raise and lower the *qi*, and how to work the macrocosmic orbit. Others suggest the method of guarding certain acupoints with rapt attention. In short, inappropriate methods abound.

To be honest, these methods have nothing to do with meditation and forming the pill. If one practices the methods by randomly copying them from a book, it could easily spur what Chinese Medicine refers to as "vacuous heat" and "evil heat," which lead to numerous illnesses. This sort of odd phenomena is not that uncommon among Daoist practitioners. This goes to show that authentic teachings are truly hard to come by.

I was once introduced by a painter who had been learning meditation from an *Yi Jing* master for many years. When I first met him, I was struck by his reddish complexion, particularly in the area between the brows. I knew something must have been done wrong. After completing the formal part of the conversation I couldn't help but ask him whether he focused his attention on the *yingtan* acupoint (glabella) during meditation. He replied in the affirmative, which confirmed my speculation. Having observed that he presented himself as a decent and genuine individual as well as a devoted practitioner, I offered a few suggestions on the issues that were bothering him at the time: feeling dizzy and light-headed, bloodshot eyes, blurry vision, excessive eye discharge, bad breath, and always thirsty.

Following my suggestions, he practiced for a while, and the next time we met he had resumed a healthy complexion.

A university professor, despite having learned meditation for a long while, found himself limited by his practice. He often suffered from lower back pain and bloated stomach. Eventually unable to put up with it any longer, he came to me to seek advice on other meditation methods. I asked him a few questions on his meditation practice and soon realized that his method was problematic, which resulted in some health issues around his digestive system and kidneys. This is highly risky in the absence of a qualified teacher who can guide the practitioner by providing correct instructions on how to circulate the *qi* along the channels in concert with in- and out-breaths. All in all, when it comes to meditation, guarding the acupoints, circulating *qi* along the eight channels, or forming the pill, the number of disciples my Daoist master taught the pithy instructions to were no more than three. These people had all previously followed and attended to the master for more than a decade. They came from good families whose wealth was accumulated only through virtuous means, possessed high moral quality, and were free from the worldly pursuit of fame and riches. [On this note] my master once shared with me some of his own experiences on how to judge character by observing subtle behavior. These, however, are not supposed to be shared with unqualified individuals. I have benefited greatly from these teachings, which I abide by till this day.

CHAPTER 32

Jiang Weiqiao's Meditation Manual—A Stepping Stone for Beginners

Zhang Yuanji was a lay practitioner from the Minnan area of Fujian province who came to Taiwan early on and had a sincere connection with my master. Because I saw him many times at *sifu*'s residence, I considered him to be one of my elders and knew that he meditated and guarded the *dantian* from early on when he was studying in Shanghai and had an opportunity to learn meditation with Jiang Weiqiao (also called Yin Shizi). Jiang Weiqiao was a notable and upstanding intellectual of the modern era who held strong opinions on education, and had in his early years studied both Buddhism and Daoism extensively. He had also established intimate friendships with the likes of Cai Yuanpei and other out-standing individuals of the intelligentsia at that time. Jiang Weiqiao always held heartfelt, passionate, and idealistic views regarding Chinese education, and therefore he and other such scholars such as Zhang Yuanji edited various school textbooks. That the famous etymological dictionary *Ci Yuan* could be completed and published was thanks in no small part to his great contributions. In particular, during his time in the commercial press (in Beijing) he edited and compiled a large collection of books that greatly influenced later generations. During the whole lengthy time that Cai Yuanpei was Minister of Education, he relied heavily on Jian Weiqiao and hired him to take charge of an important think tank that would draft educational proposals and reforms.

Owing to poor health in childhood, Jiang Weiqiao developed

a fervent interest in health cultivation, meditation, *qigong*, and other such pursuits. He maintained a lifelong devotion to meditation lasting about 60 or 70 years. Furthermore, he would go on to publish his thoughts and insights in the book *The Meditation Methods of Yin Shizi*. In those days, the lay practitioner Zhang Yuanji emphasized that it was reading this book that gave rise to his intense desire to learn meditation. Later, by chance or destiny, he got to know Jiang Weiqiao and benefited from hearing about many of his experiences regarding health cultivation and meditation. Zhang Yuanji felt that the education of the people on these matters hadn't fully developed yet; almost all other such books then found in bookstores and on bookstands would mislead the reader into a haze of confusion and were very hard to understand. Otherwise, the books would be riddled with obscure terminology and not the hint of a structure or outline to guide the reader and help them begin their study. Only Jiang Weiqiao's book stood apart from other books on meditation. Without concealing a thing, he openly shared his years of accumulated meditation experiences and combined this with knowledge from Chinese and Western Medicine, health cultivation, and other information. The book was compiled through rigorous, meticulous investigation and extraction of the valuable elements, much like sifting through sand to find gold.

Back in those days, his book caused quite the stir, and pretty much anyone who had an interest in health cultivation owned a copy. The content is concise yet comprehensive. Furthermore, it includes simple and clear illustrations, so for beginner learners of meditation it was welcome like the Gospel.

Although the old lay practitioner Zhang and myself were poles apart in terms of age, strangely it seemed as if because we were a generation apart, every time he visited *sifu*'s residence to converse with him, he would then exchange a few sentences with myself. Sometimes he would also present me with some of the books he had collected as gifts, such as the earliest version of Jiang Weiqiao's book (cited above), which had a gray cover and was composed of handwritten calligraphic script. The whole book had already started to turn yellow and was from his earliest days in Shanghai—Zhang said it was given to him by a lay disciple of the Buddhist master Dixian. In fact, I had already read Jiang Weiqiao's book long before, but speaking with the old lay practitioner Zhang gave me a deep sense of its value as an excellent reference resource for anyone starting to learn meditation. This was despite the fact that the book doesn't really expound traditional Daoist meditation techniques. Jiang had likely been influenced earlier on by the breath-counting techniques of Japanese schools and the Tiantai school of Buddhism, as well as the *tummo* (inner fire) exercises within Vajrayana Buddhism. Therefore, when compiling the book, he included many sagely tips and insights based on his own experience. Apparently, the year the book first appeared, even the great masters Hongyi and Taixu, as well as many others, gave the book their highest praise and believed it to be of benefit to the Chinese people's health and health maintenance. At that time, Jiang Weiqiao carried the book with him and traveled widely, freely offering guidance and instruction on meditation. It caught on quickly, and soon became a craze. The Shanghai government invited him many times to teach the scientific approach to meditation he proposed.

Regarding other related books, Jiang Weiqiao continued, over time, to publish many of his personal insights and experiences based on his later contact with the "Six Subtle *Dharma* Doors"[1] method of meditation as well as Vajrayana energetic methods.

In fact, during the time Jiang started learning about meditation, he relied on his own willpower, perseverance, and untiring diligence, without anyone to guide him. By finding his own way, he slowly recuperated from his previous health conditions such as lung disease and related problems (e.g., his chronic cough). He gained remarkable physical strength and went from only progressing with great difficulty to being able to happily walk ten flights of stairs and clamber up mountains. He gained from his

---

1   佛教六妙法門 (*Fojiao Liumiao Famen*): A book by the Tiantai master Chih-i that explains a six-step meditation method to bring about transcendence of suffering and purification of the mind.

own experience a deep appreciation for the benefits of meditation. Before long, he would feel a warm flow circulating around the abdomen, making the area swell and buzz. Over time this vibrating energy became more intense, to the point even that his whole body would sway back and forth completely out of his control. Later on, this wave of energy opened up his sacral region and shot up to the apex of his head. He remained in this state for a whole week before the effects finally started to wane slightly. At the time when the lay practitioner Zhang and myself talked about this, we both felt that if beginners progressed rapidly with great diligence, then actually these effects were quite normal and were nothing to worry about. However, Jiang had no one to guide him and despite this, persevered onward with no apprehension at all. That really is quite an achievement and may perhaps be owing to his personal karmic history with Daoism.

Thanks to this, he quite miraculously used meditation to sweep away all of his previous chronic ailments and even recovered from tuberculosis without any medicine. This only further strengthened his resolve and perseverance regarding the practice of meditation. From looking at the descriptive notes he made in his diary after continuing with meditation, we can see that the various states that arose, and all of his mental, physical, inner and outer experiences, were all regular manifestations of meditation practice. This includes the warm flow around the *dantian*, which later increased in strength and intensity, and even includes the energy flowing to the apex of his head (such feelings around the head are a regular phenomenon resulting from the micro- and macrocosmic orbit practice). Much like a blind cat chancing upon a dead mouse, after clearly feeling the flow go round the body a few times, Jiang fortuitously realized the feeling of carefree happiness that follows the opening of the governing and conceptual channels, and the opening of the eight extraordinary channels. According to practitioners of lore, were it not for someone being profoundly blessed with great virtue, this realization would be simply impossible to achieve on one's own. We both had a deep feeling of admiration, yet both of us shared the same view: although the book is good, one needs to keep consulting other sources while learning from Jiang's journey through these experiences while in the process of meditating. In particular, his willpower, persistence, and the diligence he applied to this practice are worthy of emulation. With these few points in mind, this book is absolutely a valuable contribution to all.

CHAPTER 33

REGULATE THE BREATH WITH RAPT ATTENTION, WITHOUT ADDING OR SUBTRACTING ANYTHING

Elder Zhang's breadth of learning was formidable; he even drew up a whole set of pith instructions dedicated entirely to meditation. Over the past few decades of his meditation practice, as he put it, he was able to gradually forgo the rigid rules and have an entirely free hand in his practice. He also once commented on how easy it was for a practitioner nowadays seeking to study the Dao to encounter false teachers rather than qualified ones—one should definitely exercise caution in this matter! He himself once spent more than a dozen *liang*[1] of a gold bar to formally become apprenticed to a master in Shanghai, only to pick up superficial knowledge he already knew. I admire him for the fact that he nevertheless expressed gratitude toward this teacher. Had he not squandered a good sum of money, how could he have learned to distinguish true teachings from false ones? This type of attitude toward learning is worthy of being followed by later generations.

Over the years that I interacted with Elder Zhang, he always treated me with sincerity and earnestly recounted his experiences to me. He explained that he was not fond of being someone's teacher, though a lot of young people followed him during his stay in Taiwan. He showed little interest in making any comments about that. To this day I still feel immensely grateful toward this elder, who has

---

1   兩: A traditional unit of weight, equivalent to 50 grams. Thus, the investment was roughly US$30,000+ as of today's value.

now passed on. Over the years, Elder Zhang left me with thousands upon thousands of words about the personal experiences he recounted, ranging from fundamental meditation techniques to the whole process of self-actualization of forming the pill. To wit: begin with the regular breath-regulation exercise, correcting posture and breathing naturally till eventually it becomes so fine that it's almost non-existent. Concentrate the mind and focus the intention on the *dantian*. Couple this method with the in- and out-breaths till you neither forget about the breath, nor follow it too closely. According to Elder Zhang, the key to a solid foundation of meditation lies in focusing raptly on the inhalations and exhalations. When the mind is focused on the *dantian*, it is called "rapt attention," whereas when the *qi* is centered in the *dantian*, it is called "breath regulation." When the mind is empty, free from delusive thoughts, and clear as a full moon, this is "not subtracting," while the state of mind that is independent from any forms of attachment, much like air in the universe, is referred to as "not adding."

To meditate, one must first adjust the mind. If the mind is still full of thoughts, make sure your eyes remain open. Keep regulating the breath till you are free from delusive thought, then keep your eyes half-closed. At this point, your mind should gradually collect and enter stillness. Then, regulate your breath and slowly meld it with the mind, until eventually you should be able to remain "raptly focused within emptiness." Retain this state of uninterrupted stillness till you achieve a state "beyond both subject and object"—a state the Daoists call "amidst the far and indistinct." During this time, true *qi* arises, but pay no heed to it; instead, continue focusing on the breath and bring it to the *dantian* to abide there. Naturally, achievement comes without force. Make sure your mind is as relaxed and open as possible, never too taut, much as you would when adjusting the strings on a *guqin*.[2] When the mind is soft and supple, it is referred to as "gentle flame"; when the mind is neither

---

2 古琴: Traditional Chinese seven-string musical instrument, whose history goes back roughly 5,000 years. It is the chosen instrument of many of the sages of Chinese lore.

tight nor loose but simply in a natural, neutral state, the "strong flame" will naturally arise. Only those with extensive experience in this field are able to harmonize and refine both the gentle and strong to the state of oneness, in order to skillfully make use of it.

During the many years I interacted with Elder Zhang, I came to understand that beginners of meditation ought to try their best to treat everything they hear, see, and perceive as if they were deaf and blind, and the mind had ceased to exist. Once this foundational exercise is solid, one's breathing will reach the level of a turtle's.[3] This is the stage where the practitioner's mind is calm, their spirit at ease. The mind of those who have reached this stage rests at all times in a most natural state—they are as if tipsy, rarely feeling bothered. A continuous flow of warmth between the kidneys may be experienced: Elder Zhang advised that one should not become attached to it, and simply let it pass. This piece of advice is of paramount importance. Despite being rather new to the practice, many worry day and night that they may go terribly astray during their meditation. This is a rather acute case of overcorrection. During meditation, if your mind is not hindered by the chaotic thoughts that arise, there need be no concern over such things as "being possessed by unhealthy influences." If you have yet to see the mere shadow of *yang* and *yin* spirit in your cultivation, the "demons" of practice will not even show their nose to you. This is quite simply overthinking, and one should definitely pursue one's meditation without further deliberation. Elder Zhang would often remind us that all that one sees is dead in essence, and that while meditating, the eyes should be regarded as simply eyes. What one ought to diligently work on instead is the spirit of the eyes, which is the primordial spirit. The first thing the fetus develops in the uterus is indeed the eyes. Similarly, when one is about to die and enter the *bardo*,[4] vision is the first sense to dissipate. While you engage in

---

3   A reference to "turtle breathing," or "fetal breathing," whereby breath and *qi* are no longer absorbed through the mouth or nose.

4   In Buddhism, the "intermediate state" between death and rebirth, during which one's consciousness/soul will pick its subsequent rebirth in one of the six realms of *saṃsāra*.

everyday activities, be it walking or sitting, never part from "a place of stillness with the two *qi*." Nourish your spirit in noisy places, while fostering your essence in quiet ones. Keep the mind still, free of delusive thoughts to cultivate your *qi*. When these three treasures are gathered as one, practitioners will naturally break through the "three gates"—namely the *weilu*, *jiaji*, and *yuzhen* acupoints.

A fellow practitioner surnamed Chen had abandoned his meditation practice for a while because of a relationship issue, and found himself in very low spirits. He asked Elder Zhang for advice, and the latter bluntly replied: "When the mind's ape is firmly held, one will not spill one's essence. When the intention's horse is tied tight, one's nature will shine bright. When one lacks the aspiration to go beyond worldly concerns or the mind to attain the Dao, alternating between diligent and lazy spells in one's practice, when one is unable to abstain from passions and sexual desire, failing to tame the mind—well, it will be impossible for sitting meditation to bear any fruit."

CHAPTER 34

ABSTAIN FROM CLINGING, AND THE ULTIMATE ELIXIR WILL COALESCE

Elder Zhang often spoke of the way of meditation. For example, he advised cultivating an unburdened mind, free of all matters—this is true regulation of the breath. When the mind no longer contains even a single thought, then you will naturally achieve authentic breathing, and you will be free from internal chaos. Spirit and *qi* will join harmoniously as a matter of course, and your mind will not waver. The three treasures of essence, *qi*, and spirit will remain stable throughout the day and night, and practitioners will naturally let loose of clinging. Spirit and *qi* will not encounter disturbances, and the ultimate goal of Daoist practice will gradually take shape. The mind without concerns, the body without action, the spirit without obscurity—if you cultivate these states long term, purified *qi* will flow without hindrance. People often speak about the "myriad levels of achievement," but none of them are able to guard, control, or cut off [lustful] desire. Being able to avoid any leakage of essence defines the level of one's attainment. The ancients said that *dan*—the mystical elixir that is the ultimate goal of Daoist "immortality" practice—begins to take form after three years without leakage; after six years without any emission of vital substance, the *dan* coalesces; after nine years, thoughts cease to arise, and all flavors become like wax. Indefatigable practice to this point will result in achievement of the golden elixir. Another note on the matter of leakage: there is true leakage and fake leakage. But after all is said and done, the most important is for the practitioner to achieve true realization and true emptiness. This realization alone can lead one to truly live without leaking precious vitality. At this point, all of emptiness is indeed the true body; it merges completely with the true body. The Great Dao, then, is near.

Lin Yanghe was an adherent to the same Daoist teachings as Elder Zhang. One day, Lin sought Elder Zhang's wisdom regarding Daoist practices for refining essence. Elder Zhang was straightforward in his advice. To relay it simply, all essence leakage stems from emotion and desire. Emotion and desire, in turn, stem from what is taken in through the eyes and thought of in the mind. If you understand how to return to lucid consciousness, then you will naturally cease to leak essence. If, for a period of time, you generally avoid leakage, then you should understand how to properly guard and circulate your full store of essence. For this practice, it is usually best to understand Daoist breath regulation. When you regulate the breath, your mouth will fill with enzyme-rich saliva, at which point you should practice swishing it around your mouth with your tongue, before swallowing it. When this is done with a balanced mind and stable qi, the full essence will be transformed. Wait until it has fully integrated into the qi channels, and then go on a relaxed walk. After 100 steps, meditate. Regulate the breath, and concentrate the spirit. During this meditation, both hands should be clenched into fists; the tongue should push against the upper gums; and you should inhale effortlessly through the nose. Use focused attention, rather than physical effort, throughout this process. After practicing this method for a short period of time, your qi will not be prone to scatter. When the qi has comprehensively circulated, relax your whole body and lie down. This is a simple and convenient practice for those times when you know your essence is full. But to ensure safety, you should only engage in this process under the guidance of an experienced teacher.

Elder Zhang gave an exhaustive account of all the possible states that might arise in Daoist cultivation, beginning with his own experiences when he was new to Daoist study. He addressed the Daoist practices of guarding and cultivating the *dan*/elixir, as well as how to restore a body that has been weakened from leakage, and how to gather *qi* in the *dantian.* In transmitting this knowledge, he strongly and repeatedly emphasized that these matters should not be carelessly shared with the wrong people; if one has not been under the examination of a master teacher for many years, and has not observed the appropriate ascetic disciplines, truly, that person should not cavalierly discuss these matters!

He then continued, addressing how to transport *qi* within the body as well as the experiences that may accompany its passage through each area. He spoke about the specific sensation associated with the passage of *qi* through the two kidneys, during which the practitioner should repress their dynamic *qi* to prevent unintentional leakage. On this part of the route, the *qi* will move through the so-called "Magpie Bridge" (the area near the palate); if dynamic *qi* is insufficient at this point in the process, it will be impossible to move the *qi* through the entirety of the body. In that case, you must wait for an opportune moment to try again. Sometimes you may be able to achieve full passage on the first attempt, and at other times you may have to send the *qi* through the process many times. The whole matter depends on whether you can sustain the movement throughout each area, and, in truth, it all comes down to the method you use to connect through three points in particular. Elder Zhang's discussion of this method was extremely detailed and concise, making the method clear so that there would be absolutely no danger in its practice.

Elder Zhang also explained the phenomenon of spiritual emergence. He addressed questions related to nourishment of the spirit fetus and described the experiences associated with the fruition of this process. He also spoke about where the practitioner should fix their attention within their body, and how and to where they should move that attention during the period of spiritual nourishment. Here, Master Zhang gave a particularly strong warning: when he had reached this place in his practice over the years, his vision extended great distances, and he could see all things with great clarity. At this point in one's practice, certain supernatural powers would be obtained, allowing one to master anything without having to learn it—this is the most dangerous area of practice. Once reaching this place, the practitioner can easily succumb to hallucinations that may arise during meditation. The key is to let go of everything, to meddle with nothing.

Elder Zhang had mastered the teachings of the *Zhou Yi*[1] and referenced this work frequently in his study of classic texts on Daoist inner alchemy. He frequently exhorted his younger followers to meditate and to consult the classic texts on cultivation, which he said were the most essential aid to Daoist practice. He said that from a young age he began deriving great benefit from Zhang Ziyang's *Wuzhen Pian*.[2] Among the Daoist immortals who inherited the Way, Honorable Master Zhang is a critical figure. From a young age, he exhibited an affinity for the study of Confucianism, Buddhism, and Daoism. When he was a bit older, he moved deeper into the study of the five metaphysical arts: mental and physical cultivation in the mountains, medicine, divination, destiny, and physiognomy. He also became a master of the *Zhou Yi*, and he would often use hexagrams to illustrate certain cryptic concepts in his annotations on Daoist inner alchemy texts. Central to Zhang Ziyang's ideology throughout his life was the importance of cultivating both character and destiny, and the transmission of teachings regarding this cultivation. He saw the human body as a vessel for Daoist practice. He even used his own essence and *qi* as medicine and transformed his spirit into internal fire. After he had received oral teachings from his teacher, he would implement them in cultivation practice, day and night. Thus, he achieved internal coherence of essence, *qi*, and spirit, and he attained the ultimate goal of becoming a Daoist immortal.

This process had a very clear, easy-to-follow order, from the foundation in meditation to the return to the void and unity with

---

1 周易: Another name for the *Yi Jing* (literally, "the changes of the Zhou Dynasty"), referring to the period the text was composed, between the 11th and 8th century BCE.
2 悟真篇: A classic on Daoist inner alchemy, composed by Zhang Ziyang in 1075. Its title can roughly be translated as *Folios on Awakening to Reality*.

the Dao. The progression required a cycle of practice, correction, and refinement. Master Zhang had the disposition of a monk, but in order to bring about the Dao more effectively, he began to practice the Daoist Way in worldly society. Because he was totally independent in thought and action, he did not have to limit himself to the company of other Daoist immortals—it is said that there were many monks of great achievement among Master Zhang's close friends. There is a story involving a certain famous enlightened master from the Chan school: One day, when they were together, the Chan master suggested they leave the location of their bodies by supernatural powers and bring back flowers plucked in Yangzhou as evidence. In the end, the Chan master's hands were empty; only Zhang Ziyang held the stem of a single, tender flower, still fresh with dew. Perfectly at ease, he stood playing with the bloom. The Chan master, having issued the challenge himself, was overcome with shame, and he realized that the Honorable Master Zhang was no ordinary Daoist immortal. Thereafter, the disciples attending to Zhang Ziyang asked him, "Why was it, if the other teacher went on the same journey, that only Master Zhang was able to pick a flower?"

Zhang Ziyang replied to his disciples by saying, "My entire life I have held fast to the principle of life–destiny dual cultivation. I practiced this truth earnestly, never daring to loosen my focus. Thus, early on, I achieved liberation through the golden elixir. At any moment, I can gather my *qi* and turn it into form, dispersing it as vapor *qi*. There is no place where I cannot take form through *qi*. Considering that, picking a flower is just a small feat. What's so mysterious about it?"

In addition to penning *Wuzhen Pian*, Zhang Ziyang also wrote *Jindan Sibaizi* (*400 Words on the Golden Elixir*). Elder Zhang noted that Wei Boyang's *Cantong Qi*, and the Daoist classics written by Zhang Ziyang, were essential reading. After Zhang Ziyang achieved the goal of internal alchemy, he upheld the mission of not transmitting teachings to the wrong people. In his life, he had been misguided a few times in whom he taught, and in each instance he encountered grave misfortunes as a result. In the last of these disastrous situations, Shi Tai came to Zhang Ziyang's aid, and in return Master Zhang taught Shi Tai the main ideas of internal alchemy. Eventually, the two of them, together with Bai Yuchan and others, came to be recognized as the Five Southern Patriarchs. Zhang Ziyang lived on this Earth for nearly 100 years before he passed into immortality. His disciples cremated his body and retrieved innumerable holy relics of all sizes from the flames.

Over the course of Zhang Ziyang's lifelong cultivation practice, he experienced countless hardships, but by the time he was 86, he had fulfilled his karmic quota for good deeds done in secret, causing blessedness and virtue to be restored to his earthly life. Owing to this, he had the good fortune of meeting Immortal Liu Haichan, who passed on to him a secret technique regarding cultivation of the golden elixir. For the next seven years, Zhang Ziyang practiced diligently according to Liu Haichan's teaching, and thus arrived at full realization of the Dao. He then recorded the quintessential facets of his life in a book. By that time, Zhang Ziyang was already 94 years old.

CHAPTER 35

Elder Zhang's Guidance on the Beginnings of Daoist Study

Sifu and the venerable scholars and Daoist elders in his acquaintance circle left behind a legacy as lofty as that of the Venerable Zhang of lore, yet they were modest in all their ways. With a quiet, unassuming air, they instructed their disciples. I and their other humble pupils came to see that these individuals and their teachings, though understated in appearance, were priceless treasures, and that their example on the path of study was truly precious. Elder Zhang based his teachings on his own path of study, speaking tirelessly of the process. Listening to these teachings, it was evident that he held boundless wisdom in the depths of his being. If one had to summarize, the most essential teachings from all the years of learning that Elder Zhang passed on amounted to just a few key steps: in his methods and practice of cultivation, he focused on relinquishing form to nurture *qi* and gather the medicine, relinquishing *qi* to concentrate spirit, and then realizing the goal of the *dan*/elixir. The ultimate phases are then relinquishing spirit and returning to void—spirit then re-emerges, and the final stage is returning to, and merging with, the void.

Among their Daoist followers, there was a retired military official who was over 60 years old. This man asked Elder Zhang how he could address the enfeeblement of the body and supplement vitality. Elder Zhang laughed and replied: "Make efforts to eat warming foods and sleep more. This is a suitable method. You shouldn't assume that you can simply make up deficits by meditation.

Many people of advanced age who begin meditating don't get very far into the practice before they are overcome with drowsiness. In this case, it is more important to make time for sufficient rest than to meditate. Once you have slept well and thus nurtured your spirit, then reconsider meditation. Otherwise, it's useless to speak more of meditation practice."

Another seeker, about 20 years older than me, spoke to Elder Zhang: "When meditating, is it more suitable to close one's eyes or keep them open? I do not understand the difference."

Elder Zhang replied: "The regular practice is to close one's eyes and assume a sitting posture for meditation. If a practitioner has not been meditating very long and isn't yet generating dynamic *qi*, then soon after they close their eyes to begin meditating, they will begin to feel sleepy. This is because the unrefined *qi* in their bodies has not yet been purified. Those who are new to meditation who are in this situation should avoid forming bad habits; otherwise, they will face extra difficulties making necessary changes going forward. Those who are relatively young should do their utmost to sit erect from their tailbone up and focus on inhaling and exhaling, aligning their mind with their breath. The body should remain as unmoving as the stones of Mount Tai, and the intention should be as still as a cold pond as geese fly over. The mind should be free of all worries. After encountering some matter, your mind and body should not be moved by any immediate changes or impulses. You should naturally enter meditation, and after some time, return to observation of the situation. The moment is then ripe with fated opportunity; the Great Dao is within reach. This old fellow himself has a method suitable for people living in the present time. First, as soon as you set out to begin meditating, you must understand all of the terminology related to internal alchemy. After you have fully understood the interpretation of these terms, they will become just like the common language of modern people. With this foundation in place, you can turn to the practice of generating warm *qi* in your lower abdomen, and your mind will feel joyful and buzzed, as if you were slightly drunk. This is one of the pleasant results when internal water and fire come together. From this point, proceed step by step, and do not waver in your perseverance. This process does not require physical exertion. Within your natural state you will enter the macrocosmic and microcosmic orbits, at which point you will be near to the way of 'fetal breathing.' From China to Taiwan, this old fellow has guided many people through these steps, and all have progressed naturally, without contrived effort, through the method of breath regulation. In this way, safely and without anxiety, they have achieved the desired results."

Yet another of the Daoist seekers gathered there was a man in his early 50s, surnamed Zhuo, who was in charge of a factory that manufactured wine bottles. He had studied meditation with *sifu* for over ten years, and he meditated upwards of one or two hours nearly every day. Mr. Zhuo would often share with the other students what he had gleaned from his study and practice. He did so on this occasion as well, bringing up matters that he encountered during meditation, which he presented to Elder Zhang. For example, Mr. Zhuo noted that as soon as he entered meditation, it seemed as if he no longer inhaled or exhaled, and when he reached this point where the breath ceased to exist, he perceived a gathering of authentic *qi* vigorously moving around his *dantian*. He said the feeling was as if a warm river of milk was flowing through him and winding around the *dantian* area, and sometimes it continued for a long time without dispersing. According to Mr. Zhou, he frequently experienced this phenomenon after practicing the macrocosmic and microcosmic orbits, and he wondered whether it indicated some sort of obstruction. When Mr. Zhou had finished speaking, Elder Zhang's face held neither a trace of approval nor surprise. With only the slightest smile, he told the man that this was a very common experience for people practicing meditation who had reached a certain plateau, and that the matter did not require further understanding. He advised the man to keep meditating.

Daoist brother Zhuo then continued to ask Elder Zhang questions related to "fetal breathing." Zhuo said that after he meditated, he always felt a rogue strain of breath circulating in the area below his heart and above his navel, sometimes rising to the crown of his head, or sliding down to his *yongquan* points. He remarked that when this happened, his whole mind and body were often overcome with a carefree, exuberant feeling, and he wished that he were able to dwell in that state and preserve the sensation more often. However, he felt unsure as to whether doing so would be correct practice. Elder Zhang replied: "If there still seems to be breath flowing unceasingly, then these sensations do not comprise genuine 'turtle breathing.' For someone who has actually entered 'turtle breathing,' a piece of thin yellow paper that adheres to the nostrils upon the initial inhalation will neither fall out nor slip from its position after a prolonged period; this proves an authentic experience."

CHAPTER 36

Remain Centered, Holding Fast to One Principle—Mind and Breath Will Align

In sum, Elder Zhang's way of sharing the Daoist arts was highly accessible and clear, in contrast with traditional methods for meditation. He put special emphasis on the study of temperament and mental cultivation, as well as the principle of letting events unfold organically, without forced action. Furthermore, he required himself to perform virtuous deeds every day, storing up these merits toward enlightenment. He often remarked that if only one party benefits through instruction on the Dao, then this transmission is not very meaningful. Additionally, he emphasized that the means of modern media made the sharing of text and images extremely easy, and that most people are guilty of excess in this regard, temptations being so abundant. He often exhorted young people to avoid any kind of sexual activity once they had begun to study meditation. Furthermore, he advised those who were married or had a partner who was not a student of the Dao to take extra care to prioritize the control of their desires. He would also teach people how to calculate timing during intercourse, and he addressed a variety of other generally taboo topics—to wit, he suggested not to engage in sex while there is thunder and lightning, or when one is inebriated. He would also tell young disciples repeatedly that in the present age, it is not appropriate to pass on the "supplementary technique" of the Southern School. Elder Zhang said that the majority of the seekers he had seen who chose to study through the teachings of the Southern lineage had bad results. Consequently, he repeatedly impressed upon us young disciples never to compromise the quality of our actions and never to take advantage of other people, even people with whom we were in close relationships. Students must recognize that the only way to make progress if one follows the Southern School is to adhere closely to the sexual restrictions: the Great Dao must be pursued in emptiness, not in matters of carnal flesh. The so-called upper-level key phrase to internal cultivation is, in fact, "the preeminence of inborn vital *qi*," the realization of which emerges only from emptiness.

Elder Zhang said that the most reliable scholar of these arts was Chen Tuan, who lived as a recluse on Hua Mountain. Chen Tuan's central emphasis is captured in one sentence: "Remain centered, holding fast to one principle: mind and breath will align." This pithy phrase, unfettered by additional wasteful words, represents the quintessence of internal cultivation. Elder Zhang required us to study and practice this idea unceasingly; its usefulness is infinite.

To explain the Northern School teachings on cultivating quietude, Elder Zhang principally used the *Ling Yuan Dao Ge* (*Verses on the Origin of the Soul*) and the *Er Shi Si Dan Jue* (*24 Mantras on Internal Alchemy*). His presentation of these teachings brought on a profound sense of illumination. A certain Daoist student among those listening had been following the way of the Wuliu Sect of immortals under the Southern School for many years. At this point, he returned yet again to question Elder Zhang about "planting and collecting" techniques. Elder Zhang responded measuredly: "If they want to cultivate these arts, male practitioners must not leak any semen through the *yang* pass, and female practitioners must cease their menstruation cycle. It is apparent to me that you struggle to cut off your sexual desires and still experience leakages of essence. Therefore, it is not suitable to engage further with your question."

It was clear that the naturalness Elder Zhang espoused was to be found by keeping to a humble, pure path. Elder Zhang often said to me: "All the true secrets of these arts can be found in the

Cantong Qi; one needn't look elsewhere. Modern people are overly ambitious because they don't understand the essential teachings on internal cultivation. They think these mantras are simple, but this is a great error. People often question me regarding the Southern School cultivation practices, but the majority of those who pose such inquiries haven't attained any semblance of control over their lusts and passions. Don't they consider that these teachings are easier said than done? At the very least, female students must stop their cycle so that they will not leak any essence through menstrual blood. But this requires at least two or three years of skilled practice to accomplish. As for male students of *qi* refinement, if they want to reach a point where they avoid even the smallest leakage, they must focus on not ejaculating in their sleep, and this certainly cannot be accomplished without three years of work. These are fundamental parts of training, but it seems many people cannot master them. So, what's the point of asking so many questions? They even fail to use the 'rerouting the river chariot rotation' technique to confront erection, so there is really no point in further discussion. Incidentally, I have observed that there are a few meditation practitioners in Taiwan who do not understand the method of directing attention to the *dantian*. In any case, if they come to the point in the microcosmic orbit where heat rises, or if their *yang* ascends in the middle of the night, they simply cannot focus on anything else. This is actually a dangerous habit, which, if perpetuated, can damage the body beyond purification. One cannot be too cautious about habits related to harmful leakages."

Among *sifu*'s students was the owner of a hardware company. Before this man—who looked like an old Daoist priest—came to *sifu* for guidance in meditation, he had already studied internal cultivation elsewhere. He too asked Elder Zhang about the ideal moment to gather internal medicine. Elder Zhang replied: "When your whole body feels relaxed and warm, your four limbs are slightly numb, and saliva is continuously churning in your mouth. These indicate the most basic level of awareness, but you cannot rely wholly on this state to determine that it's time to gather internal medicine. You also need to pay attention to whether your mind holds any disturbance or unresolved issue—for example, whether sexual energies are still emerging, or whether any emotional matters are influencing you. If there is any aspect of your mind or body that is not fully quiet and pure, this also requires attention. In particular, it is critical that you bear no anger. If any anger emerges, you must wait another ten days before you revisit the possibility of gathering internal medicine. In sum, the state of one's body and mind is no simple matter, and cannot be discerned casually from ordinary books. Rather, it is best to learn under the direct guidance of an experienced teacher."

Zhang Boyu was an officer actively serving in a certain military unit. On weekends, he often came to visit *sifu* and ask questions about meditation that he encountered in his daily practice. As he happened to be visiting at the time we were gathered to learn from Elder Zhang about the myriad challenges of internal cultivation, Zhang Boyu took advantage of the seemingly fateful opportunity to ask some of his own questions: "Thinking back to when I had just begun studying meditation years ago, it seems that I actually experienced fewer illusory thoughts then. My meditation practice has since deepened, but as time went on I have found that stray thoughts have been stirred up like dust. When I meditate, my mind is flooded with illusions. At this point in my practice, how should I deal with this?"

Elder Zhang answered him: "The problems you are experiencing are very common in meditation. You have not yet mastered the art of stillness, nor of temperament cultivation. If I instructed you to extricate all the thoughts you mentioned from your mind, to focus only on letting go, you wouldn't be able to do it. Instead, I will teach you a mantra. As soon as illusory thoughts arise, just recite the mantra. When the words leave your mouth and your ears hear these sounds, your mind will follow the rise and fall of the phrases, and eventually disappear. If you recite this mantra aloud until you reach the cessation of illusory thoughts, then continue meditating. Otherwise, gather all the blood collected in your head and direct it to the *yongquan* points, then, use your hand to rub them until they feel comfortable. Another option is to smack your hands together, rub them until warm, and then massage your kidneys. Then massage down the insides and outsides of your thighs, applying enough force to create heat, until you reach the bottom of your feet. These methods can also help you dispel illusory and scattered thoughts.

"However, the most important thing is to understand how to become adept at nurturing *yang qi*. The training of *yang qi* starts in the eyes. One must become as if blind; the ears, deaf; the mouth, mute; the whole body, unmoving, as a boulder. Whether during meditation or in going about daily activities, train yourself in this way. Your spirit will gradually merge with the void, and when your *yin* reaches its extreme pole, *yang* will form. Little by little as you sit, the four limbs will become filled with vigor, and you will feel as if the blood vessels throughout your body have dilated. As you are going about your day, spend more of your free time reading the *Heart Sutra* and the *Scripture of Purity and Quiescence*. In fact, the two words, 'purity' and 'quiescence' represent the key to unblocking all of the thousands of energy gateways throughout the body; one cannot dismiss them as unimportant. In the so-called process of 'passing through the gate to enter into oneness,' all of the appearances, sounds, and other stimulations of the world are perceived as one, and this oneness is the crux to entering stillness. It is a state of endless profundity. You must constantly discipline and correct yourself in your training if you are ever to attain self-knowledge. The humble fellow before you once heard the following account of a certain old Daoist on Wudang Mountain: The old Daoist entered meditation and remained sitting for one year, at which point his Daoist brethren all thought he had died to the physical world and transcended into immortality. An experienced Daoist elder came to examine the scene and called for the postponement of cremation. Then, they took up an inverted bell from in front of the temple and, beating the instrument lightly, softly called out the sitting Daoist priest's name. He instantly responded, his eyes opening slowly. The experienced Daoist elder urged him not to speak, lest he harm his *qi*. He instructed him how to massage and manipulate his four limbs and the posture of his body. When he began meditating, this Daoist priest's handle on the Daoist arts can be summed up in the concept of 'quiescence.' Indeed, all mastery of the arts arises from attaining profound stillness and maintaining the optimal state of the *dantian*."

CHAPTER 37

THE BENEVOLENT TEACHER'S INSTRUCTIONS ON HOW TO GRASP THE TRUTH OF THE DAO

Though dozens of years have passed since the time I spent in *sifu*'s residence, I can still describe the impression it left. It's as if the residence's mosaic inlay has been permanently set into my own heart. Where his home used to stand, now yet another high-rise has been built. In former times, the grounds were filled with the sound of voices reading and reciting sacred texts, and there were dragonflies and butterflies chasing each other through the garden. In the summertime, all was a profusion of blooms and colors. The fragrance of osmanthus was all-enveloping, and two or three Daoist seekers would be reclining under the 100-year-old banyan tree, enjoying the cool shade and discussing theories of the Dao. Only Xiao Gang's verses can truly conjure the feeling such a scene evoked:

> In a wide-open garden, dusk falls and mist rises
> Without burden, unbound and solitary, I have not yet thought
> of return.
> The tall willows hide behind a veil of green,
> Red lotus flowers gently part the water's cover.
> Swallowtail butterflies, wing after wing,
> A pair, soaring in unison above the flowers.
> Each understands the language of the other,
> Of one mind, never to separate.

Originally, these lines were meant as a metaphorical description of a man and woman united in heart and mind until the end of time. But in those days of study under *sifu*'s roof, we Daoist seekers were like blood brothers: the closeness of our emotional bonds was even stronger than that of siblings. Even after so many years, I am still in contact with some of my fellow disciples from that time.

Sifu's abode was home to a vast number of butterflies. There were even some that a senior apprentice who had studied biology at National Taiwan University couldn't identify. One of the most common sightings was the golden birdwing, which is relatively famous among the butterflies of Taiwan. Its wings are a mix of a thrilling gold and mysterious black; to see it dance in flight among flowering shrubs is truly stirring. The *daimio tethys* [in Chinese, the "jade-belted butterfly"] was also abundant. The entire abdomen of this butterfly appears to be a deep black-brown, but when it spreads its wings to fly, it reveals a beautiful white stripe across its belly, almost like apron springs. There were also many lemon emigrants: according to the disciple who had studied biology, lemon emigrants' bodies change color in accordance with the vicissitudes of climate and temperature. One moment they are white, and the next they are grey—a true marvel! If you have a chance, you can observe this transformation for yourselves.

On several occasions, *sifu* stood upon a tatami mat laid out in front of the French windows and, gazing upon the many colorful wings dancing through the flower bushes, relayed the butterfly dream story from the *Zhuangzi*. It exactly reflected our ultimate goal in meditation: to become one with the natural order. *Sifu* also used this classic parable to teach us how to distinguish between reality and illusions, that we might not be misled by sensual pleasures. Butterflies both put people at ease and spark their sense of intrigue. The poets have consistently turned to them as objects for verse.

The poet Li Shangyin scrutinized some ancient Daoist classics on the art of internal cultivation. Eventually, with quite a solipsistic posture toward the whole matter, he decided that he should follow the example of *Zhuangzi*, and was thus inspired to pen the following poem:

> *I wonder why my inlaid harp has fifty strings,*
> *Each with its flower-like fret an interval of youth.*
> *The sage Zhuangzi is day-dreaming, bewitched by butterflies,*
> *The spring-heart of Emperor Wang is crying in a cuckoo,*
> *Mermen weep their pearly tears down a moon-green sea,*
> *Blue fields are breathing their jade to the sun…*
> *And a moment that ought to have lasted forever*
> *Has come and gone before I knew.*

These lines quite aptly capture the memories of my youthful years. At *sifu*'s residence, at once so stately and leisurely, we basked in our studies. And now, just as Li Shangyin describes, the light of the present shines on these things of the past as they settle into beautiful recollections.

From my boyhood through the prime of my adult life, I immersed myself in wide-ranging study of Daoism, Confucianism, and Buddhism, shedding all ambitions. In that Daoist enclave in particular, I never felt the tug of worldly pursuits, and I developed an extraordinary sense of renunciation. The visitors at *sifu*'s residence were all erudite scholars who arrived wearing simple cotton clothes with leather belts. Most of them were masters who carried themselves with an elegance worthy of study. These were formative impressions for my young mind. My sights weren't set on great fame or prodigious ambition. In fact, what I envisioned for the future was to have a dwelling by a hill with a small stream out front, idle clouds floating overhead, a pool of clear water to enjoy, and a small pavilion atop the hill. The house would be bright and clean, with two or three paintings and a *guqin* hanging on the wall. I would bathe in the fragrance of incense made of Chinese cedar kindled in its burner while sipping tea served in porcelain cups. A pair of cranes would be walking slowly along a peaceful path in the garden, and some Daoist friends would trail behind them. There would be no candles in front of the flowers, and pine trees would provide plentiful firewood.

Amid discussions of the Dao, if I began to feel sleepy I would simply use the *guqin* as a pillow. The passage of time in the outside world would be of no consequence—I would simply observe that when the flowers opened, spring had arrived, and when they fell, autumn had ended. Life would be utterly devoid of striving. I would pay no attention to the vicissitudes of worldly tastes. I would only meditate, with old books and oil lamps as my companions, and in this way I would be perfectly content. Although this was a fool's dream, at least it was not founded upon the fantastical illusions of human affairs.

A scroll of calligraphy, painted with bold strokes, hung from the left-hand-side windowsill in *sifu*'s entryway. The skill behind this piece was quite fine; the characters radiated a special energy. The piece was signed Wu Yuanzi. I still clearly remember the few lines of text:

> Reject sensual pursuits to cultivate a calm mind. Meditate often to collect your thoughts. Guard your disposition by ridding yourself of all corruption and lust. Use the ancient maxims to protect your consciousness. Enlightenment will come through understanding the intrinsic order of one's nature.

These five sentences were constantly on my mind back then; they wouldn't leave me alone. Of course, this wasn't some sort of ground-shattering axiom that leads one to a sudden breakthrough, but they are critical reminders for Daoists practicing the ways of meditation and internal cultivation.

Later, I learned that Wu Yuanzi was an accomplished Daoist and an ancestor of the lineage. During the Qing Dynasty, he was a critical leader in the School of Complete Reality. He also wrote several books, such as *Uncovering the Truth in the Book of Changes* and *Teachings on the Wuzhen Pian*, which contain invaluable contributions to our knowledge of meditation and internal cultivation. In his path toward enlightenment, he emphasized to all the disciples he instructed that they must never waver in their adherence to the principles of dual cultivation for nature and fate. He wanted his successors to meditate and not to be hasty or covetous about achieving new skills or reaching higher levels of practice. Students must follow the proper sequence in training if they are to grasp the critical principles of internal and external alchemy. Wu Yuanzi's many written works elucidate that the process known as "gathering medicine" is to be carried out within one's own body, and that *qi* is to be collected from the void. He was extremely focused on the theories of *The Book of Changes*. His understanding of the work is clear in his writings on the *Cantong Qi* and the *Wuzhen Pian*. His annotations on these texts are undeniably effective: he guides readers to the root of the concepts. Many people have benefited from the benevolent gift of his written teachings. It is no wonder, then, that *sifu* often spoke admiringly of Elder Wu during teachings on the *Cantong Qi*.

It is said that Wu Yuanzi was motivated to begin practicing Daoism after falling ill. For the rest of his life, he was highly disciplined in his practice of the traditional Daoist arts for cultivating longevity—eventually, he achieved the ultimate goal of internal cultivation. At the end of his days, this great teacher broke through all doubts and became enlightened, leaving behind his elderly body to become an immortal.

In the early days of the meditation class, *sifu* would invariably weave stories of the ancient immortals into his teachings. He encouraged and cautioned our generation of disciples through accounts of our predecessors seeking the Dao and facing evil spirits in the process. He most admired Lu Chunyang (also known as Lu Dongbin), one of the Eight Immortals. Apparently, from childhood, even before he had begun to study the Dao, *sifu* read *Tales of the Eight Immortals*. He was most compelled by the account of Lu Chunyang learning the way of the Dao from Zhong Liquan. Legend has it that Zhong and Lu encountered each other in an old drinking parlor in Chang'an, and Lu Dongbin was initially intrigued by Zhong Liquan's peculiar mode of dress and general appearance. Shortly thereafter, Lu was stunned to see a poem that Zhong had written on the wall—the immortal destinies of Lu and Zhong had fused. Zhong Liquan was aware early on that Lu was no ordinary fellow, but that he had not yet found the correct path, and thus persisted in worldly habits and was fettered by evil obstacles. Zhong asked Lu to write a poem, and when Zhong read the verses Lu had penned, he nodded his head knowingly. He already recognized the beginning of a fated bond between them. Zhong artfully sent Lu into a dream state, and in Lu's short dream, a microcosm of his whole life unfolded.

Everything unfolded lucidly: Lu passed the provincial exams in his youth, brought honor to his family, went to the capital to take the civil service exams, and was named the top scholar in the land. The emperor doted on him, and this attention also sparked notice of the prime minister's daughter, a breathtakingly beautiful young woman. She and Lu were a perfect match, and they passed happy, devoted days together amid the successes of Lu's career as a government official. Lu basked in his meteoric rise. But just as he had reached this lofty, seemingly untouchable point, his beloved wife contracted an incurable disease. She died, leaving behind Lu and their two young children. Lu remarried shortly thereafter. His second wife was the wealthiest noblewoman in the kingdom. Their chemistry was immediately apparent, and they quickly formed a strong connection. Children were born one after another, and they all exhibited promise for civil and military vocations. For the moment, Lu's authority covered the kingdom. In the court, he was second only to the emperor in power; if Lu commanded it, it was done. But ten years of this good fortune passed in a flash, and the emperor passed away. His successor had long ago begun to take issue with Lu Dongbin. Now that this new emperor had taken up the throne, how could Lu avoid being targeted? Before long, the emperor set a devious trap for Lu, falsely charging him of wrongdoing, and sentenced him to exile in the wilderness. Lu was exposed to great snobbery and was scorned by all. As he was being escorted to his desolate destination, he experienced myriad bizarre and painful events, and became overwhelmed with grief to the point of wanting to cut his life short. As his will to carry on was slipping away and his heart sinking with heaviness, the smell of fresh rice suddenly wafted into his nostrils, and he awoke. Lu let out a tremendous sigh of relief—it was all just a dream!

Zhong Liquan laughed as he observed Lu Dongbin awakening from the dream world. He limited his speech to guidance, speaking only words of instruction. Lu Dongbin was a man of wisdom, after all, so he had surmised that Zhong Liquan had had something to do with this dream. Zhong, still smiling, said to him: "What you have experienced is something that almost all living beings pass through. Consider your life. Your middle-aged years have already come to an end. In this later stage of whatever time you have left, don't you want to have a plan?"

It was as if Lu Dongbin had been struck by lightning. Now fully alert, he quickly kneeled before Zhong Liquan: "This disciple has realized that you, sir, are a great teacher. Please accept me as your follower from this day forward and guide me down the correct path. I beseech you, transmit the way of the Dao to your humble student, that I might yet have a chance to accumulate merits and virtues."

Zhong Liquan was, after all, a Daoist immortal. He subjected Lu Dongbin to an examination to determine whether Lu had truly relinquished his attachment to the world and was ready to seek the Dao. In total, ten trials were set before Lu Dongbin. One by one, he passed the tests, but Zhong Liquan did not immediately begin transmitting the Dao to him upon these successes. Rather, the immortal would give Lu a few of the classic Daoists texts and instruct him to read them with utmost care. Lu Dongbin was required to study these materials on their own; and each time, Zhong only gave him fragments, a few phrases here and there, and then he would depart, as elusive as a wandering cloud.

Finally, Zhong Liquan decided to transmit the Dao to Lu Dongbin. He opened their conversation with these words: "On the path toward enlightenment, Daoist practitioners must be alert to ten demons, which they will certainly encounter—the demon of affection, the demon of the six senses, the demon of female charms, the demon of wealth and honor, the demon of sainthood, the demon of the six emotions, the demon of material goods and profit, the demon of war, the demon of adversity, and the demon of licentious female entertainers—as well as nine types of danger. That is, sometimes, in the name of pursuing the Dao, you will find yourself poverty stricken and overwhelmed with problems, passing some nights with nothing to eat. You will encounter creditors from past lives who have come to demand justice, entangling you in emotional debts. You may also come into fame and fortune and find yourself blinded by a desire to gain more, or find yourself afflicted with any of the many possible internal or external afflictions of the physical body. You might encounter a confused teacher who misguides you, or inexplicable, contradictory discussions and schools of thought in which you are utterly at a loss for clarity. On the path of Daoist cultivation, it is difficult to avoid seasons of confusion, disorder, restlessness, and weakened resolve, which will all delay your progress in attaining the Dao. Additionally, if these experiences result in the formation of bad habits, you won't be able to regain control of your circumstances. You will come to feel as if your head is on fire, and you have no means of dousing the flames. The worst fate of all would be separation from peace and prosperity, to run hither and thither and not be able to access the means of settling your mind, meditating, and practicing internal cultivation toward enlightenment in the Dao."

Thus, Zhong Liquan gently outlined to Lu Dongbin all that one might experience in body and in mind, internally and externally, on the journey toward awakening to the Dao. He laid out all of the most common psychological, spiritual, and material trials of this process.

These are just a few brief scenes from the fated relationship between Zhong Liquan and Lu Dongbin. Of course, teacher and disciple subsequently had many predestined exchanges, and Lu went on to overcome innumerable obstacles, challenges of a sort that an ordinary person would find impossible to manage. Thus, Lu earned Zhong's guidance—a great honor which Zhong never bestowed lightly—and the teacher proceeded to transmit to him many spiritual treasures and instructed him in the way of the immortals.

CHAPTER 38

RELEASE YOUR GRIP ON FATE, CULTIVATE HAPPINESS AND WISDOM

Personal affairs and property are often fretted over in the name of reputation.
While meditating, summon your concentration and survey worldly affairs.
Human plans are far inferior to the destinies laid out by Heaven.
The scheming mind is always striving. The Daoist mind is calm.
Everything of yesterday proves fickle and is cause for doubt.
Arising from a night's sleep is like rebirth into a new reality.
When you speak with a wise person, their [quality of mind] will be apparent.
A foolish person is also easy to identify.
The affairs of this world are like a boat with a short sail;
It may glide toward western or eastern shores, under many cycles of the moon, with numerous winds from the south and just as many from the north.
Everything is impermanent. A person's passage into old age has no bearing upon the beauty of spring or how many times the flowers blossom.
When you hear of quarrels and other human affairs, you must recognize them for what they are, but play deaf and dumb to them.
But when you do act, it should be informed by intuition and conscience, with deliberation of right and wrong. A person should never act carelessly or in a confused state of mind!

What can you say today of [the warlord] Xiang Yu [who ended his life in the] Wu River?
And who inherited the lot of Zhou Yu from the Battle of Red Cliffs?
Where is the satisfaction in victory?
There's no shame in letting others [have their way].
Over worldly matters, people could struggle endlessly with one another.
[Better to] offer a friendly face and avoid a dispute.
New buds open on the branch that, last year, dropped dead flowers.
Dwelling on bygone days of youth can put you in a stupor.
White hairs, now many, seem to urge you on toward death.
No amount of gold can buy back the prime of life.
That some magic medicine could halt the aging process is wishful thinking.
Sorrow wells up with the recognition that no rope can fasten you to this moment.
These sentiments should not be discussed with your descendants; wait until they experience old age for themselves.
Throughout the human world, there is endless chaos. Even if you lived forever, you would not be able to make sense of it all.
The body you are attached to—who will know of its transient existence years hence?
You can make a thousand years' worth of plans, but when you die, all your schemes will disappear.
The sun rises and sets. Time cycles along, and you cannot hold it down.
It flows like water; it will not reverse course.
People who remain stuck in worldliness do not understand the Will of Heaven.
They stay up worrying throughout the night for nothing.

This widely known poem was written by gifted scholar Tang Bohu of the Ming Dynasty. It is Tang's attempt to awaken his readers, inviting them to learn from his own experiences living a dramatic and constrained life. Naturally, one cannot mention Tang Bohu without another famous Ming Dynasty literatus coming to mind: the famous novelist Feng Menglong. My own curiosity about Feng Menglong was actually sparked back by the film *Flirting Scholar*.[1] In the Ming era, Feng Menglong's literary genius was highly esteemed. He was not only famous as a novelist, but as a literary scholar more broadly and as the author of several famous operas. When I was in school, I read his works *Stories to Awaken the World* and *Stories Old and New* several times, in addition to his *Chronicles of the Eastern Zhou Kingdoms*.

Once, at an elder's house, I serendipitously picked up *The Life Story of Wang Yangming*, which Feng wrote in the latter half of the Ming Dynasty. It was because of this text that I came upon Feng's nickname "Old Bearded Man." Many academics have debated this book over the generations, but these scholarly disputes are beside the point. First and foremost, this work captures the spirit of Wang Yangming; it is distinctive among all books of the time in which he is represented. The book was an invaluable contribution to Ming-era literature. If I may also note, the average person can give an in-depth, animated description of Tang Bohu but is prone to overlook the great extent to which his destiny was intertwined with Wang Yangming's. Wang Yangming was not only a powerful politician and military strategist; he had a critical influence on Chinese culture as a whole, shaping Chinese art and education. Especially notable among his accomplishments was that within just one month he completely quashed the rebellion of the Prince of Ning. The Prince of Ning had worked on his scheme for over half his life, but in one stroke Wang destroyed the traitor's plans and wiped out his stronghold of power.

Not least among Wang's admirable qualities is that he was devoted

---

1　唐伯虎點秋香 (*Tang Bohu Dian Qiu Xiang*): A famous Hong Kong comedy movie directed by Stephen Chow, from 1993. The title and stories are based on Feng Menglong's fictionalized stories centering on Tang Bohu, the famous Ming painter who lived a century before Feng.

to the plight of all common people. There are few such people who don't hesitate to risk their own glory on behalf of the greater good. Through his lifelong demonstration of benevolence, Wang was the savior of people throughout the Jiangxi region. He spoke without reservation; in the name of truth, he offended many important Confucian scholars. He also offended the extremely famous Zhu Xi. I often think that if Wang Yangming had lived just a little longer and been able to guide a greater number of students, later generations would more clearly understand the principles of his critical work *Chuan Xi Lu* (*Instructions for Practical Living*). The *Chuan Xi Lu* primarily comprises a record of Wang Yangming's candid words among his students and various people in similar circles. The text is worthy of exploration, especially for students of Daoism and meditation. A thorough reading is extremely beneficial for understanding the mind and temperament. When we fail to achieve a state of stillness in meditation, the most important factors are the inability to attain internal peace of mind and the inability to dispel external seductions. In such a state, there is no way to merge one's essential nature with one's greater being. Wang also emphasizes and offers a unique perspective on how to cultivate a blameless private life, maintaining vigilance when it comes to observing the mind even when one is alone—the virtues of which we discussed previously.

There is more to be said about Wang Yangming and Tang Bohu's predestined fortunes. The two were actually schoolmates, but change dealt with their lives quite differently. Along with Shen Zhou, Wen Zhiming, and Chou Ying, Tang Bohu came to be known as one of the four great masters of the Ming Dynasty. Those who understand Ming Dynasty novels and history will recognize that *Flirting Scholar* is a false representation of Tang. In total, Tang Bohu was married three times, and each of these wives had nothing to do with Autumn Fragrance, Tang's love pursuit in the popular story. The historical Autumn Fragrance lived in a brothel in the city of Nanjing and was the most celebrated courtesan of her time.

A certain period of Tang Bohu's life was riddled with difficulty and grief. When he was still a young man, his father, wife, mother, and younger sister, with whom he had a very close bond, all died in quick succession. Of his originally large family, only he and his younger brother remained. Ultimately, the challenge of overcoming these experiences may have become his engine. After studying intensely for a year, he earned the top score in the provincial examination. He also excelled in poetry and painting. His creative work was highly regarded throughout the scholarly class and wider society as a whole. His name was known and esteemed in the imperial court and beyond. However, Tang Bohu's official career was not all smooth sailing. At one point, he was framed for a crime and thrown into prison. After this incident, he lost interest in the world of official positions and fortune, and turned to seek contentment among the famous mountains of lore. He began interacting more with the literati of Jiangnan and Jiangbei, and he came into contact with many senior monks and venerable elders from Buddhist and Daoist circles.

Widely respected scholars in the Qing Dynasty were the first to publish critiques of the errors in *Flirting Scholar*. The true identity behind the male protagonist who pursued Autumn Fragrance was said to be the debonair young scholar Chen Yuanchao of Suzhou. Following the circulation of this discovery, people finally realized that Feng Menglong had fabricated the novel's storyline of the male hero marrying the famous concubine. Leaving aside arguments regarding the stories and characters in his writings, I have indeed read most of Feng Menglong's oeuvre. Among the works I've read is *Extensive Records of the Taiping Era*, which Feng wrote in his later years. Judging from the various recorded accounts of him, I was most impressed that Feng didn't just write novels—he managed to quietly make benevolent contributions to society and accrue virtues. He offered piercing critiques of the chaos and injustices surrounding him, inciting revolutionary change. For example, a widespread practice at that time was for families to abandon or drown newborn girls. Feng Menglong considered this phenomenon wholly tragic, cruel, and without humanity. Consequently, he composed "Drowning Girls Is Prohibited: An Announcement" for his book. The essay forbids female infanticide and is directed toward all members of society. Because of this subtle, virtuous act, innumerable female lives were spared.

However Feng Menglong is remembered in history, I have begun to regard him as unique among the literati of his day. In that closed, narrow-minded world, he was early to recognize the dignity of women, to encourage them to hold their heads high and live lives of honor. This view permeated his essays as well as his works of popular fiction, in which the value of female life was demonstrated through his female characters. His propagation of these progressive ideals is deeply admirable.

In sum, from the process through which immortals attained the Dao, to the written works of historical figures, the same principle is evident: in order to reach enlightenment and become an immortal, one must accumulate merits and good works; and, even more importantly, let go of all preconceived notions of cause, effect, and destiny. Those who meditate should not just sit stubbornly in boredom; one must cultivate wisdom and happiness to transcend the strenuousness of practice and gain internal medicine. All that is thought of as good or evil can be said to stem from the mind. If one has a benevolent mind, then the benevolence will come to fruition through the person, and they will be enveloped by a spirit of good fortune. Those devoted to accumulating virtue through good works act benevolently without the desire for recognition. Gradually, these charitable deeds accrue and manifold blessings return to the doer, filling them with satisfaction. Not only that, but all calamities and curses are dispelled from their lives.

Practitioners of Daoist internal cultivation and meditation must never perform evil acts. They must bear a mind of benevolence and mercy, loyalty to their country, respect for their parents, and fraternal love for their compatriots. They should continually correct and refine themselves, use benevolence to transform others, go to the aid of those in crisis, take pity on the poor, enjoy the joys of life, and avoid jealousy. They must not undervalue others, nor hold an inflated opinion of themselves. If others insult them, they should bear it without resentment; and if they are overly praised, they should feel a quiet sense of shame. They should give alms without expectation of repayment. In general, they should give material goods to other people without any hesitation, not clinging to anything. If they want to enjoy longevity, they must do a minimum of 1,300 good deeds. Furthermore, even tiny acts of goodness are important—such opportunities should not be overlooked. Killing and bringing any harm to the life of sentient beings are the greatest injuries to virtue. You should not disturb any bird or beast or living creature, much less trap animals in their burrows or abort fetuses.

To rejoice in a person's death, to speak ill of a person's greatness, to hide a person's virtue, to wastefully consume a person's capital and assets, to sow discord among one's kin, to act as an accomplice for evil, to threaten a person's security and blessings, to ruin a person's fate, to be heartless in pursuit of wealth, to act traitorously in the name of business, to lessen a person's strengths, to protect one's own shortcomings, to thwart good or kind behaviors, to wish ruin on someone upon observing their wealth and good fortune, to entertain lustful thoughts when confronted with someone's physical beauty, to harbor resentment over things one cannot attain, to mock a person's appearance, to envy a person's ability, to look upon one's wise teacher with anger, to be unfilial toward one's parents, to indulge in drink and licentiousness, to engage in violence against one's own people, for men to be disloyal or dishonest, for women to lack gentleness, to be irreverent toward the spirits of one's ancestors, to go against one's elders… In a word, all of the reliable instructive texts contain clear warnings: the practice of meditation and internal cultivation is more serious than common affairs. The practitioner must be aware that in following this path, they call the attention of the spirit world onto their person and will be subject to inspection. Light offenses may be punished with days whittled from one's life; heavy offenses may be punished with injuries of the body and health, even disaster upon one's descendants. If one has done any sort of evil deed, one must repent and do whatever is required to change one's ways. Then, only after a long period of time, one's lot will shift from disaster to blessing. These teachings must not be ignored.

CHAPTER 39

CONCENTRATE THE SPIRIT ON REFLECTING ILLUMINATION— REFINE THE SPIRIT TO BECOME ONE WITH THE VOID

The Daoist elders from whom I have learned about the Way all emphasized the centrality of mental cultivation. Various immortal ancestors began training in Confucian and Daoist cultivation before beginning their formal pursuits of the Dao. Such conditioning is based in the traditional teachings: maintain a pious and deferential internal life, practice self-restraint and propriety. The masters all advise that a seeker first focus on becoming an upright person. If a disciple fails to act with humanity, then it is of no use for them to spend long periods sitting in meditation. A person who tries to attain transcendence without confronting these foundational matters cannot become a sage, much less achieve immortality!

On my own path, all of the Daoist immortals and elders I studied adhered to this principle: that is, that seekers of the Way must begin by achieving full humanity. Only by first mastering the human way can one connect with the heavenly way, and transcend worldliness. Everyone who meditates and practices Daoist cultivation must do so in total purity, adhering to the principle of non-action, maintaining inner tranquility, not striving for anything but rather returning to their unadulterated self.

Those who have just begun to study the Dao should remember to read aloud from the *Dao De Jing,* the *Scripture of Purity and Quiescence*, and other teachings on calming the mind and on non-action. The purpose of this practice is for the student to achieve a mental state as vast as the universe, and to be unfettered by the conventions of the world. This is the precondition of connection with Heaven and Earth, of entering into communication with the universe. Elders and senior practitioners who have gained this consciousness and experienced the realm of immortality exhibit an expansive magnanimity in all their dealings and interactions with people. Their manner is as open and vast as the sea, as pleasant and accommodating as spring. Whether active or at leisure or engaged in any matter, they are always natural and smooth, totally at ease with themselves and their surroundings. Their character can only be described through comparison with the finest of weather, the brightest of days. Their comportment is unusually impressive and dignified. Whether they are giving instructions or engaged in discussion, their speech is always clear and sonorous, and they keep their bodies perfectly clean and pure, like maidens. Their disposition is noble, reflecting a mentality as clear as the moon after a storm, and their spirit exudes a greatness like that of Mount Tai among the Five Sacred Mountains. From one's first encounter with such a person, their aura of dignity and loving kindness is never not apparent, never lapsing. They are exceptionally cultured and refined, yet exist above worldly norms, invulnerable to common vulgarities. In those early days, all of the elders and masters I called upon had such presence. I began harboring private fantasies that one day I would come close to their state of being. Such were the naive dreams of my youth.

All that I gained from studying under these various masters of ages past underscores that the dual cultivation of disposition and being is essential for contemporary disciples of meditation and Daoist internal cultivation. In the present age, the highest priority should be to liberate the mind and extricate oneself from the traps of the world. The masters often said that if, in meditation, one cannot first release the myriad preconceptions and retain only breath, then no length of meditation will bear any fruit. This is very true. To speak of today's situation, many Daoists find that after meditating for years, they are yet to make any progress in the Daoist arts.

The main reason for this is that they have not disentangled their minds from the vulgar vines of the world. They can never be free of this hindrance if they persist in clinging to their many plans and preconceptions, which contribute to instability of mind and reason. It will be a great misfortune to them if they continue meditating without changing their approach.

I often say to my fellow Daoists, if you frequently calm your mind, you will begin to see lotus flowers wherever you look; if, in meditation, you probe to the root of things and fulfill your nature, all ground will become your meditation cushion. Ten years ago, I met a Taiwanese practitioner on Wutai Mountain. Most days, he worked on scholarly texts, and he always supported and promoted his juniors. He was quite diligent, working hard in all his endeavors. This fellow often commented that from the time he began meditating at a young age, he would sit for long stretches of time, often not rising from his posture through the whole night. And yet, no matter how long he sat, he was not able to empty his mental landscape. This failure to reach the void and purify his mind vexed him. One day, he came to the place where I was staying. As we discussed the matter over tea, I offered him a bit of humble advice: "The most important thing for a Daoist to avoid is obstinacy and attachment. My recommendation is that you abandon your regular routine for a few days. Spend the whole of each day enjoying flowers and bathing in fresh water, and then see where your practice stands. When you reach a certain point in meditation, it is critical that you do not get hung up on achieving a certain goal, and then find yourself stuck, overly fixated on that aim. Thus, if one day you can awaken to an experience of unified, relaxed body and mind, totally emptying yourself of thoughts and vexations, and a return of your consciousness to your true soul, to your natural alertness, then will your authentic spirit return and settle within you. Genuine meditation may manifest in later life, when you achieve stillness even during activity, and in stillness gather spirit. In everything, you will be relaxed, without contrived effort or action. In a peaceful, quiet moment, you will be able to fully appreciate the peace and quiet.

Even if you only get one instant of that feeling of tranquility, you nevertheless enjoy the lightness and grace it brings. You will no longer impose differentiations upon the various experiences you encounter, nor prescriptive ideas for how to approach them. If you can reach this state, every moment of tranquil consciousness will be like 10,000 years of meditation.

As it has been said, 1,000 cups of wine cannot compare with a single taste of peaceful water; 1,000 good grains of rice cannot compare with a single drop of sweet dew. In meditation, it is of utmost importance that before sitting you let go of all you cling to, relax, and set your mind at rest; only then will you be able to reap twice the gains with half the effort. To enclose yourself in a room devoting your hours to walking meditation and chanting to the Buddha is far better than exhausting yourself rushing through busy streets. But an entire day spent venerating the Buddha does not measure up to one moment of a quiet, clear mind. That clear consciousness is most critical of all: whether a practitioner is able to obtain the internal medicine via the slow-burning fire depends entirely on it. This presence of mind is *qi*. In this state, the practitioner's mind is like still water; the three treasures naturally cohere, and the three internal medicines are gathered without effort. Essence, spirit, and *qi* merge into a unified whole. Then the practitioner is indifferent to the differentiation and pursuit of the internal or greater cosmos, and the gathering of small and big medicine is redundant—for the golden elixir is never apart from them.

If you've read *Feng Shen Bang* (*The Investiture of the Gods*), then you know of the legends where everyone was prepared to confront Nezha's wind-and-fire wheels at any moment. If your entire consciousness assumes a limpid spirit, and you make the appropriate adjustments after your internal fire rises, then your six roots and six dusts—that is, all sensory organs and the stimuli they receive—will merge, and every instant will extend itself to you as an opportune moment to gather big medicine; even more so, the middle hour of the night, about which you will harbor no illusions. Internal and external realms will be laid bare, merging together, and so too the Ten Directions will have no boundaries between them. Once you reach this point, what need is there to 'build the internal fire'? The only thing that will remain will be the illumination of nirvana—what need will you have for thinking about the *dantian*? If your spirit is concentrated on reflecting illumination 24 hours per day, then you will have no more need to practice via the governing and conception channels, because the golden elixir will form on its own, as a matter of course."

The Daoist disciple listened to all of this, and insinuated understanding and agreement, nodding his head vigorously. However I doubt that he had truly understood my explanations. The principle of meditation cannot be found on the mat. If you wish to understand it, you must apply your whole mind to unifying every reach of the universe. Ultimately, there should be no separation of internal and external, of body-spirit-mind and Heaven and Earth, of the firmament, and the entire cosmos. This is the beginning of *samādhi*[1] in meditation.

A certain number of years later, I heard from a Daoist elder that the Taiwanese Daoist had died. One winter evening, he had a fit of anger related to some family problems. During dinner, his vital blood *qi* surged. The ambulance didn't arrive in time, and he died before reaching the hospital. It was evident that the biggest challenges this practitioner faced had nothing to do with opening the three gates of the body, but rather with the external openings of fame, emotion, and wealth.

What I have been discussing will only be accessible to practitioners who have a solid foundation. For the average person who practices meditation and Daoist internal cultivation, the more salient matter, after establishing correct posture and quieting the mind, is full concentration on observing this *gongfu*. In meditation, this observation occurs when one returns to a state of attentive listening through the discipline of the outward-focused mind. The Daoist practitioner's mind is based in their eyes, ears, nose, tongue

---

1   From the Sanskrit, a "meditative absorption/mindfulness" that is non-dualistic.

[and other sense organs]. All of the six roots house our spirit. If you sense that any of these roots are leaking toward the outside world, then you should examine your mind and breath. Tune yourself to see whether thoughts are racing, *qi* is not preserved, voice and countenance are not at rest, or spirit is not peaceful. Without the cessation of thought, essence will remain deficient.

In fact, all this can be summarized in the issue of bringing one's thinking mind to a halt. Everything that has been discussed requires the cessation of thought, self-restraint, and self-refinement. When you meditate, mind and thought become interdependent and the breath returns to the navel. This process is the way to self-refinement, and to make progress, you must persevere in reflecting all light and sound until true *yang* emerges. If you have the opportunity, you should devote more time to studying the *Scripture of Purity and Quiescence*, which will have a great effect on your practice. Gradually, internal heat will dissipate, and the waters of the kidneys will rise. This is the moment of harmony among the internal elements. Over time, the ultimate goal will be achieved. But what I'm speaking of here is only the beginning of the process. To refine your spirit, you will yet have to adjust the authentic breath until no air flows through your nostrils, no thoughts arise in your mind, and you have severed your ego and gained awareness of spirit. Through ongoing regulation, when you reach a point where this restful state of mind never disappears, and where spirit and *qi* are unobstructed, the principle of "growing old with unfailing eyes and ears" will be realized. All substances that circulate will be in motion along their proper courses, and medicine will be gathered. After the internal fire, you can deliberate upon internal fluctuations, and when these adjustments have been completed, you will finally have an opportunity to move closer toward the void.

All progress in meditation practice depends on whether, upon sitting, the practitioner is able to cut themselves off from the many currents of disturbance, putting up a veil and deflecting any stimuli from the outside world. They must focus entirely on the critical acupoints, and authentic *qi* will move through them naturally.

Then they will be able to execute the "five vital breaths oriented to the origin."[2] Finally, if they can realize the emergence of activity from extreme stillness and stillness at the apex of activity, they will understand that they must completely release both, deflecting all stimuli of the six roots. They will return to a unified breath as the only imperative.

---

2   五氣朝元 (*wu qi chao yuan*): A very advanced stage of inner alchemy, in which the *qi* of all internal organs is able to coalesce instead of being scattered.

CHAPTER 40

RID YOURSELF OF ABSURD THINKING, RETURN TO TRUTH THROUGH THE DAOIST ARTS

Modern people are physically busy and mentally strained. Therefore, I don't recommend they use the ancient masters' methods of guarding the critical orifices and acupoints. Rather, if practitioners are able, they should apply their greatest effort to aligning mind and breath through techniques based in the six sensory organs. For example, when the eyelids are half shut, if whatever the eyes see excites the mind, immediately return your sensory attention to the breath. Focus entirely on the incoming and outgoing breath until the mind reaches a state of stillness. If the ears, through taking in all sounds, cause division or chaos of the mind, then you should immediately return to the breath. Again, gather your whole attention and fix it on inhaling and exhaling, continuing to adjust until you have achieved total calm. If the nose takes in some common smell that you like, and this produces illusory thoughts, at once, move your focus to the breath, following the same method of complete concentration on the inhalation and exhalation. During meditation, if the body and its contact with the external world produce internal reactions and illusory thoughts in response to any manner of sensation, including soreness, pain, itchiness, numbness, swelling, coolness, heat, dryness, or moisture, then this also requires a prompt shift of attention to the breath as it comes and goes, until the mind is placid.

From top to bottom, your entire body must be thoroughly relaxed in your sitting posture. Sit, then, until your physical form, the great void, and Heaven and Earth meld into one. Sit until both person and method vanish, self and material world are empty, and you enter the natural wholeness of all that exists. Access to what the Daoists refer to as the "golden elixir" depends on the foundational ability to enter the void and gain mystical longevity.

As is written in the *Dao De Jing*, "Man takes his law from the Earth; the Earth takes its law from Heaven; Heaven takes its law from the Dao. The law of the Dao is its being what it is." The most critical idea is the last sentence, this phrase about the natural way of things. This is the most important concept for Daoist cultivation practices. The practices of the macrocosmic and microcosmic orbits, the method of "transporting the celestial chariot," and the timing of nourishing and warming practices are all measures to address discrepancies in the capacity of practitioners. Some of these exercises are primarily for restoring the collection of *yin* and *yang*; some guide accumulation of *yin* and engagement in good works; some rely preliminarily on proactivity and later introduce non-action. To sum up, there are innumerable methods for cultivation, and each practitioner must determine their individual path according to the fate they carry from their past lives and their inclinations in their present one.

In my humble opinion, all Daoist practice is rooted in the principle set forth by Laozi and Wei Boyang. From this insight, one can get a sense of the whole picture. No matter how difficult the label or form of a method, or how abstruse the contents of Daoist scripture, in the end, one must always return to excising illusions and pursuing original truth. This is the only method by which one can enter the realm of complete reality. Along the way, the seeker will inevitably face all manner of setbacks, but it is precisely through these challenges that they will be able to understand the meaning of returning to the original substance and fulfilling the mission of being, to concentrate wholly on reaching a yielding, soft existence and merging with the void. However, even if—through practice—you reach a state of unified radiance with all things, it still falls under the category of methods that Laozi referred to as "formed through causes and conditions" [as opposed to *wuwei*, non-action, free from causes and conditions]. The average practitioner who has been performing cultivation exercises for ten years, sometimes longer, has experienced all the methods of the internal furnace, used intention to gather medicine, created warmth and nourishment through adherence to the early morning cycle of *gongfu*, and facilitated the emergence of *yin* and *yang* spirit. However, these practices are merely convenient stop-gap measures for lack of alternative means of reaching the ultimate goal. Wise practitioners who have a natural gift for Daoist attainment, after having practiced cultivation, all understand that the body is the furnace, and the mind the bright room of awareness. They combine this understanding with stillness in meditation, relying on the natural circuits to create internal fire, "increasing and reducing fire," avoiding restless thoughts while guiding *qi* at the proper hours, and adjusting and nourishing mind and breath. They concentrate their whole attentive capacity into a unified whole, and through spiritual trance, they reform themselves. They can gather as spirit or disperse as pure *qi*, and are thereby able to transport themselves through shifts of form, coming and going from their bodily selves at will; their spirits manifest as their beings. And then, how do they live? And what about when one still has not realized the six paths of Daoism, access to many locations, arrival at the station of the immortal, enjoyment of karmic blessings? Furthermore, is it not true that after receiving karmic blessings, the karmic cycle is such that hardship will follow? These are all points of inquiry that I struggled to understand and brought before my elders and masters for many years.

If you have a masterful teacher to guide you early on in your studies of Daoist cultivation, the effects of your practice will be evident within a short period of time. Your mind and body will lighten, chronic ailments will dissipate, and you won't have any nightmares. You will even be able to practice Daoist *bigu*[1] fasting, no longer requiring meals. Many Daoist disciples' experiences reflect these transformations.

Many years ago, I met with an old Daoist, originally from Guangdong, who was living in Xinzhuang. We were fated to meet several times. Upon these encounters, I noticed that his coloring slightly resembled beeswax, and he emitted a slight glow, like a halo. His eyes lacked the fogginess evident in most older people's. The scleras were pure, and the irises shone with the deep color and vitality of a child's. According to his disciples, by the time the old Daoist was 92 years old, he had no bottom teeth left; and then, one day, three or four new teeth suddenly grew in. At 90-something years old, he still spoke with great vim and vigor, and his memory and mental faculties were excellent. He recounted details of his Daoist studies from years past in great detail, as if all had just come to pass the previous day. When asked about specific cultivation formulas, he had all the answers at the ready, never needing to search his thoughts. Surely he had attained the Dao.

The man's disciples said he had not taken a regular meal in many years. Each day, he only drank some grain-based liquid. The disciples also said they had not heard of him catching a cold or being sick in any way for many years. From a few snatches of conversation, the main impression the old Daoist gave was that the subject of his studies was incredibly complex—he often intermingled the rhetoric of many schools of thought in his explanations. However, all taken together, what he said was quite cogent, and in fact aligned under the polemic of one school. That said, it also seemed that he was engaged in the dual study of Daoism and Buddhism. He often interspersed his speech with coded references to *Mahāmudrā* and *Dzogchen* teachings.[2]

---

1   辟穀: Literally "to refrain from grains." An advanced form of fasting practiced on the path toward immortality.

2   From the Sanskrit, literally "Great Seal" and "Great Perfection," the two highest, ultimate practices in Vajrayana/Tibetan Buddhism. They require previous completion of many preliminary practices and must be transmitted directly to the disciple by a qualified teacher.

The old practitioner had investigated the Dao throughout his life. He remarked that from the many fated realizations along this journey, his conclusion was that a seeker must forget form, forget *qi*, forget spirit, forget emptiness, and ultimately, through continued practice, even forget the word "forget," releasing the concept itself. He cautioned against becoming disembodied and playing in the spiritual realm just outside of the abandoned physical form, noting the risk of not being able to find the means of return to the form. Many people idled away or were lost to such a state, and he found this a great pity.

Once, arriving for an appointment, I happened upon the man performing the art known as "bone-shrinking," a form of contortion. In just three or four minutes, he could manipulate his body to fit entirely inside a small basket. It was a very strange and mysterious sight. He must have studied the traditional techniques of this folk art as a young man. In any case, I just mention this incidentally, those exercises not being relevant to Daoist enlightenment.

Daoist practitioners who have been successful in the practice of internal cultivation bear some marked differences from ordinary people in their physical and spiritual bearing. When I was in my twenties, I had the chance to visit Chaozhou Township in Pingtung County, where I stayed with a Daoist elder who had come to Taiwan from Sichuan. In his younger years, this master had studied meditation alongside a monk and become very skilled, even without the formal instruction of a teacher. I couldn't suppress my curiosity over this fascinating person, and I had a bad habit of digging until I got to the bottom of something. So, I boarded a train with a fellow Daoist and made the long journey to the mountainous area, which at that time was still quite poor and far removed from general society. What I admired most about the old Daoist's life there was that the main reason he had chosen this abode was to be of assistance to the impoverished indigenous people who dwelled there. He not only taught the local children how to read Chinese characters, but also used healing *qigong* arts to cure the community members' diseases. It was said that if a person fell ill, the Daoist needed only to apply his full intention to the affected area of the body and project a healing force, and most patients would respond immediately. They would feel an itching sensation and then an intense heat. In this way, mild afflictions could be healed in one session. In more serious cases, the same extraordinary results could be achieved with just three to five sessions.

You may wonder, then, just how advanced was he in the internal arts? Once, some of the indigenous people caught a wild hare and offered it to him to express their gratitude for his benevolent presence among them. When the Daoist elder saw the hare, he breathed in and then blew upon it. From that one breath, the meat was immediately roasted. The Daoist then sternly admonished the villagers to stop hunting sentient creatures, for it was counted as a karmic offense. Moreover, he instructed them to take the roasted hare into the mountains and perform a proper Buddhist burial, dedicating merits to it. The old Daoist's intention was to make the people aware of his spiritual abilities. By inspiring frightened awe in this instance, he convinced them of his power, and thus they would believe him when he spoke of the importance of not killing.

From reading the *Baopuzi* and other ancient texts on the Daoist cultivation, I had come to understand the techniques involved in these arts. The texts also differentiated between internal cultivation and external cultivation, and noted that the loftier the attainment in these cultivation practices, the greater likelihood that the practitioner could become an immortal. The descriptions of the exercises and the cultivation process included references to this type of masters of the *qi*, noting they could turn all their blood from red to white, and emit fire from their bodies. They also had the ability to send out their spirits to occupy external things. No external sensory stimulation could disturb their inner state; they could direct spiritual beings and control the forces of nature. In fact, one of the powers mentioned is the ability to burn things using *qi* expelled with the breath.

This suggests that the Daoist elder in the mountains had reached a similar plane of skill in these arts. When we met to chat, he spoke little, but from those few words I gained invaluable, boundless wisdom. I cannot express how immensely the treasures he imparted on me helped my meditation practice at that time. But the seasons change, and the months and years continue to move along. After seven or eight years, I heard from some fellow Daoists that the elder in the mountains had passed away. Considering the wealth of good deeds he built up and his cultivation practice, I have no doubt that he is now counted among the immortals.

CHAPTER 41

In Buddhism and Daoism, Understanding and Practice Hold Equal Weight

In passing, *sifu* also brought up the opportunity he once had as a youth to know an old Buddhist monk well versed in Confucianism, Buddhism, and Daoism. This monk would later become Sichuan's famous "Guanghou Monk." It was said, in addition to his keen facility in the *dharma*, he had studied Daoist internal alchemy and opened up his meridians and channels at a young age. After succeeding in the practice of inner alchemy, he took up Vajrayana Buddhism, which he mastered, and ultimately reached enlightenment. Consequently, he traveled around, picking up whatever teachings he could find.

One of the monk's students and attendants once commented that, ever since Guanghou had completed his inner alchemy, he had never seen the monk lay down in a bed. In fact, the monk's spartan room, according to the reports of his students, contained nothing more than a meditation mat. Day and night, the master applied himself ceaselessly to meditation.

In the early years of his alchemical aptitude, the Guanghou Monk often ventured to high mountain peaks, with blistering temperatures around 20–30 degrees below zero, to meditate. With a frozen, ice-slick world all around him, he would often sit for ten days at a time and forego lying down to sleep for half a month, shielded only by a single garment of clothing. During his retreats, the snow around where he sat would melt and snowflakes would evaporate before landing on his body. These were the more obvious marks of the depth of his skill. In addition, after entering meditative stillness, he would go about a month without eating or drinking, yet never feel the pangs of hunger. Even more miraculous was that, during brutally hot summer days, if others wore the same monk's robes, they would soon find themselves drenched in sweat. Monk Guanghou could, on the other hand, travel 100 miles in a day in the heat, without so much as a single bead of moisture to be found on him.

In the past, when in mainland China, *sifu*, like Monk Guanghou, had the opportunity to come into contact with Vajrayana Buddhism and subsequently made connections with many famous Buddhist masters of the time. It was just such a mutual spiritual bond that brought Monk Guanghou and my master together under the tutelage of Master Nenghai. Master Nenghai was from Sichuan and in those years he and Master Dayong (an Indian Buddhist author also known as Āryaśūra, "The Great Brave," or "Ārya the Brave") were among the earliest to study Vajrayana. After completing his studies, Master Nenghai translated a number of important Buddhist scriptures, thereby making a profound contribution to Buddhism. Due to his accomplishments in Vajrayana, he was named as one of the successors of Tsongkhapa, and held the title of *Dharma* King and holder of the Gelugpa School. He was clearly held in very high esteem.

It was thus that, through their mutual destiny with Master Nenghai, my Daoist master could come to understand the heights of Monk Guanghou's spiritual achievements.

From the Daoist perspective, only when someone has successfully mastered the internal alchemical process can they use their body's own *yang qi* to assist others through healing. This also happens to be quite dangerous and damaging to oneself. Monk Guanghou would often use his true *qi* on the acupoints of patients to treat their illnesses. For him to exert himself in such a dangerous and sacrificial way required a great deal of compassion. It was said that he had helped countless thousands of people, and that his selfless conduct and quiet virtue had already earned himself a spot amongst the highest ranks of immortals. Despite this, Monk Guanghou went to abnormally great lengths to keep himself out of the limelight. Wherever he went, even if it was to assist others, he would never leave behind his given name, surname or even his Daoist name.

The old master was undoubtedly proficient in medicine and acupoints, and well versed in acupuncture, otherwise it would have been impossible for him to navigate the various points along the pathways of the governing and conception vessels during the healing process. With great precision and ease, he was able to bring heat to any point along the eight extraordinary meridians simply through touch. He sometimes worked so quickly that he could treat over 100 patients in one session.

From everything my Daoist *sifu* told me of Monk Guanghou's incredible conduct, what I admired most was the immenseness of his mind. It was like peering out over the spot where a river pours out into the broad, borderless sea. There was nobody in the past 100 years who could have stood shoulder to shoulder with him. What brings me to these comparisons? In a world where many become pigeonholed by the dogmas that arise from their school or sect, Monk Guanghou's students said that he repeatedly urged them to learn widely and listen far. He warned them not to get mixed up in any system that presented narrow and stagnant views. He also promoted an all-embracing approach toward Buddhism and Daoism. He held great respect for, and excelled in, Chan Buddhism, whether it was the Linji, Caodong, Guiyang, Yunmen, or Fayan Schools. However, he did not blindly stick to traditions and customs but rather took the affairs of everyday life as starting points to help people learn; nor did he lay too much emphasis on complex distinctions which would entangle people and leave them lost as to which course to follow.

According to many of the senior monks who had met him in the past, Guanghou had an incredible familiarity with all the pithy instructions of the Daoist path and was able to both understand

and carry them out in practice. Although at that time there were numerous people who sought teachings from him, and his name was known widely, he never took advantage of any of these connections for personal agendas or gain. He also wouldn't get into debates about rights and wrongs with people, and kept a modest demeanor.

What a great loss it is that, at present, not a single written line or work [by him] has been found to pass to later generations. Not only that, but in his later years, this incredible master was said to have met his end at the hands of a fellow practitioner, just as he was determining to go beyond mortality and into focused retreat.[1] Master Nenghai most likely had an inkling that Guanghou would encounter this misfortune, and although he had helped him make all arrangements for his retreat, in the end there was nothing he could do [to help Guanghou avoid his fate]. We can only hopelessly resign ourselves to the fruition of some predestined karmic retribution! Thus, this great monk's time in the world came to an end.

In Daoism, practitioners will invariably come across oral tips regarding Daoist inner alchemy to be done after they complete the meditation phase of their practice. If we speak strictly of the teachings as passed down from the ancient masters, modern people would find them very difficult to practice. The most supreme teaching is, in fact, still centered on the mind and coming to regard the space of the entire universe as the cauldron for creating the golden elixir (pill of immortality). One's inner mind is already complete, and one should rely on the sky as the basis for creating the pill, pure practice and non-action, and being free of any impediment. These form the soil out of which the golden elixir of internal alchemy is created. The spirit and body become the alchemist's lead and mercury; meditative stillness and wisdom become the pathways for the alchemist's water and fire; stilling the mind and quelling delusive thoughts become the alchemist's form of bathing; discipline, meditation, and wisdom are the most vital of all the

---

1   閉關 (*biguan*): An individual practitioner engaging in focused practice in seclusion.

alchemist's elements. Ultimately, your practice ascends until the distinction is lost between the spiritual and the physical form. One goes beyond the physical form, and this and internal spirit alike are transformed into something miraculous.

At that time, when I read the works of the realized Daoist Li Daochun from the Song Dynasty, I was shocked and awed at how closely his life's practice and works resembled the teachings of the Buddha and how much of his work shimmered with the marks of Chan. If a person were not proficient in both the Northern and Southern schools and did not thoroughly understand *chanji*,[2] how could they reach such a state? From this, one can understand that if a Daoist practitioner wishes to truly become realized, aside from learning from the world as if from a great teacher, it's also paramount that they have an experience of the Nature of the Dao. If one blindly pursues and becomes attached to physical cultivation, to "gathering the medicine," to regulating fine and coarse breath, no matter if one distills the elixir and melds one's spirit with the Dao, if one remains attached to one's views, one could meditate for a hundred years and it would all be in vain.

2　禪機 (*chanji*): The subtle mystic environment created between the teacher and student that functions as a medium for further spiritual development.

CHAPTER 42

LI BAI'S FORGETFUL TENDENCIES ENDING HIS CAREER AS AN OFFICIAL

Li Bai was in his early forties when he was granted special favor from the emperor, a gesture perceived as an indicator that his political career would see rapid promotion without further efforts. But what the poet lacked was an acute sense of how political power worked in the imperial court. Just when his career was about to take off, it came to an abrupt halt when he encountered his karmic creditors. His poetic genius was highly appraised by Emperor Xuanzong of the Tang Dynasty, who repeatedly invited him to drink and recite poetry at court. The celebrated "Song of Serene Melody," an ode to Lady Yang Guifei [Emperor Xuanzong's favorite concubine] is one such example of Li Bai's talent.

Despite his literary genius, Li Bai did have a small personality flaw: when he started drinking, he would forget where he was and what he said. In addition, the part of his personality that paid no heed to trifling formality would expose itself in his dealings with people on such occasions, which inevitably offended others. If the people he offended were true gentlemen, then all would be fine; however; Li Bai had unwittingly offended two of the most influential, yet uncivilized, people at court. If he had only asked Yang Guozhong to prepare the ink [to write his poem], it would not have been a big deal. Unfortunately, he also demanded that the powerful eunuch Gao Lishi remove his shoes. After that, the desire for revenge against Li Bai became deeply rooted in Gao's heart.

Gao Lishi had been looking for opportunities to avenge himself on Li Bai and now the poem "Song of Serene Melody" presented itself as a perfect excuse. He claimed that a section of the poem concerning Zhao Feiyan, the favorite concubine of Emperor Cheng of Han, contained mocking metaphors and hinted that she was lowly and lewd.

In fact, Lady Yang and Zhao Feiyan didn't share much in common in terms of either their upbringing or later experiences. Zhao's grandfather was a famous craftsman of musical instruments. Her father also learnt the trade from his own father who was also adept at fixing, tuning, inventing, and making instruments. He later found his passion in composing and singing his own music, gaining fame and popularity that far surpassed the crafts tradition handed down in the family.

Due to his natural talents in musical performances and his advanced singing techniques, over time he started to receive invitations from government officials and notable statesmen to perform at parties in their homes. Eventually his talent was recognized by Zhao Man, a lieutenant from the city of Jiangdu, who became a big fan. Zhao Man would often invite Feng Wanjin, Zhao Feiyan's biological father, to have dinner with him and family. The frequency of his visits eventually led to Zhao's wife falling for him and, after a secret affair, she became pregnant. The embarrassing thing was that Zhao Man was sterile and therefore unable to get his wife pregnant. How could she explain the sudden change in her appearance? She excused herself to stay at her parents' home during her pregnancy, and from there she made a deal with Feng that since the child was his own, he would raise the child, yet the child was not to take his surname but would rather go by the family name Zhao. To this Feng could only nod his assent and the child later became known as Zhao Feiyan. Zhao Feiyan later transformed into a beautiful young lady, winning everyone's hearts in the family. She was also extremely bright and had such an outstanding memory that she almost never forgot anything she read or heard about. No matter whether it was in terms of her countenance, her physique or her complexion, she was well above the average girls of that time.

Born into a family of adept craftsmen with a musical tradition, Zhao Feiyan was skilled in calligraphy from a young age. She was particularly good at singing, was very eloquent, and a people pleaser. Since she wasn't the biological daughter of Feng's wife, she had a rather laissez-faire upbringing, an experience that eventually led to her having an unruly personality and restless, showy nature. As she was good at being on everyone's good side, she naturally gathered scores of suitors. If one were to write a book on her romantic liaisons, they would be too numerous to even be listed.

Her first love was a young officer of the imperial guard with whom she formerly had relations. But later Zhao Feiyan was able to earn the affections of Emperor Cheng, charming him, and attending to him obediently. Ever since winning his favor, Emperor Cheng never turned to another within the imperial harem. Due to overly engaging in debauchery in his everyday life, he was already aged, and his vigor declining, while Zhao Feiyan was in her prime, like a flower in full bloom, so how could she be satisfied? It was said that in private she had affairs with so many male attendants that waited on her that there was almost no one left with whom she had not had secret romantic liaisons. This Emperor Cheng was also quite strange. He was clearly aware of Zhao Feiyan's promiscuity in the court but felt helpless. Even more ridiculous was that he would punish any person who informed him of her adultery. Furthermore, Zhao Feiyan also had a little sister named Zhao Zhaoyi, who also earned the favor of Emperor Cheng. It was said that later, Emperor Cheng came down with a most taboo dysfunction in the men's department. But strangely, if he even touched Zhao Zhaoyi, then the issue would be resolved and he would be "as good as new." This led Emperor Cheng to dote on her even more. Later, when it came to the cause of Emperor Cheng's death, the outside world said that he died on Zhao Zhaoyi's bed. But the true reason was that the previous night, when the two were frolicking about, after Zhao Zhaoyi had had too much to drink, she accidentally gave Emperor Cheng seven stimulant pills, and in the end he became overstimulated and died in her arms. Numerous are the historical descriptions of the Zhao clan, but there is no way to verify their veracity; because they were preposterous and incredibly obscene, they could not become part of the official historical record, and thus were passed down to later generations through operas and novels instead.

Of course, Yang Guifei was very aware of Zhao Feiyan's reputation in the eyes of ordinary people and after hearing Gao Lishi's explanation of Li Bai's poem, she felt a great sense of disgust toward Li Bai. Because of this, whenever Tang Xuanzong wanted to give Li Bai a promotion, the process would be secretly blocked and interrupted by Yang Guifei. From that time onwards, Li Bai's political career was in tatters, even to the point that he became exiled when he was still in his prime. Although Li Bai had been gifted with original literary and artistic talent, he was accustomed to being unrestrained and doing things his own way, so given that he also could not contribute his talents to the kingdom, he started to wander the land and went among the hills and by the sea. On his travels he even forged some connections with Buddhist monks and Daoist priests.

CHAPTER 43

TRUE IMMORTAL HIGH WIND, INDIFFERENT ATTAINMENT OF THE ROOT

In the Tang Dynasty poems, there are ten infamous immortal companions, the head of which was Sima Chengzhen. Among the ten, Li Bai felt a close affinity with, and an enormous amount of admiration for, Chengzhen, revering him like a deity. Li Bai himself once said that in his early twenties he had felt utterly fascinated with him. After they met in person, Chengzhen had felt strongly that the youth before his eyes was of uncommon temperament, excellent artistic ability, and held the manner of someone who had seen through the trappings of the mundane world. After exchanging only a few words, Chengzhen praised Li Bai's high potential. Li Bai had made a deep impression.

Li Bai as well felt the need to express his admiration for Sima Chengzhen, later writing a piece called "Ode to the Encounter between Peng and the Rare Bird," in which he described how tremendously heartening the praise given to him by Chengzhen had been. The encouragement had awakened Li Bai's dormant creativity, and by means of these poetic tributes, he was able to pay respect to Chengzhen's magnanimity as well as his own heart's desire to follow him. What long-lasting significance and influence, then, did Chengzhen impart to later generations of Daoist practitioners?

Sima Chengzhen is a legend in both Chinese and Daoist history. At one point in his life, he lived and practiced in seclusion on Tiantai Mountain in a place called Tong Bai Guan. During his cultivation in quietude, he dismissed all outside affairs, but his reputation nonetheless spread forth, even reaching Empress Wu Zetian and Emperor Ruizong. Chengzhen received many invitations to the royal court to give lectures and sermons, the most famous of which is a short story about a question-and-answer dialogue between him and the emperor.

Since the emperor was sincerely reverent toward Daoism, and because he knew Sima Chengzhen had already achieved the level of an immortal, Ruizong always waited on and treated him as a national treasure. Ruizong had from an early age been fascinated with the principles contained in the *Book of Changes*, and on one occasion consulted Chengzhen about a question he had concerning a certain divination technique. Chengzhen believed it unwise that the leader of a country spend his days playing with games and numbers, instead of having a broad chest and advancing his great ambition. He chose some words from the *Dao De Jing* to inspire the emperor. He told Ruizong that the heart of every man must possess certain principles. The six roots and one's innate temperament are closely related and cannot be increased or decreased. It is absolutely unnecessary to waste time studying these kinds of cunning sophistries, only adding to one's burdens. Ruizong found this teaching profound and sensible, and thus proceeded to request guidance on building character, handling worldly affairs, and governance. Chengzhen spoke plainly, saying:

> The way of a country's governance is the same as self-governance: all things should be dealt with through "non-action," a pure, clear heart, and scant desires. Hold no personal agendas or selfish motivations. Don't oppose the forces of Heaven, and follow the Natural Law. Be faithful, honest, and sincere. Then the country will naturally follow the Great Way.

Over the course of his rule, the emperor invited Sima Chengzhen to stay in his court, and Chengzhen knew that he and the emperor were acting on a connection from previous lives. Therefore, he often gave secret teachings and imparted secret Daoist incantations to Ruizong, and the two developed a close and congenial relationship.

Ruizong intended to award him an official title and allow him to stay in the palace, but Daoist immortals could not accept a salary, so Chengzhen would not comply. Ruizong respected his choice, and when the time came for him to leave the capital, the emperor chose a particularly special and beloved zither from his personal collection and gifted it to Chengzhen as a souvenir. Then a great crowd of well-wishers gathered to bid farewell, both civilian and military, and the emperor bestowed poems of farewell. This was his and Ruizong's karmically destined relationship.

Sima Chengzhen had a destined connection with several of the Tang Dynasty monarchs, such as Emperor Xuanzong, who was very reverent toward him and many times requested him to stay at the palace. But Chengzhen knew that his relationship with Xuanzong and with Ruizong were quite different. Therefore, no matter how many times Xuanzong requested secret Daoist methods, Chengzhen skillfully circumvented his attempts with a few choice words. However, Chengzhen did suggest that the emperor set up Daoist temples on the eight major sacred mountains, and Xuanzong later heartily gave permission, sending forth a "heavenly mandate" that all mountain summits and forests in the areas erect Daoist temples in hopes that the deities would bless the country with peace, prosperity, and favorable weather.

In the year that Sima Chengzhen was close to 80 years old, Emperor Xuanzong had occasion to summon him to the palace to accept offerings. Xuanzong had felt strongly that Chengzhen's hermitage on Tiantai Mountain was much too far from the capital, making visitations near impossible. With all sincerity and piety, Xuanzong offered Chengzhen his choice of a secret temple on Wangwu Mountain, not far from the capital. After this secret monastic retreat had been constructed, Xuanzong personally wrote the calligraphy signboard for it. Not only this, he also sent his younger sisters, princess Yu Zhen and Wei Di, to go and serve Chengzhen and study his great teachings. Since then, Wangwu Mountain has become an historically significant and extremely cherished paradise.

According to Daoist historical records, Sima Chengzhen be-came accomplished in internal alchemy at a young age, and was also exceptionally gifted in *daoyin* and the techniques of health cul-tivation. It was not surprising that he was able to live an abnormally long life, until he was well over 100 years old. What's more, his face held no traces of age, and was as lustrous as a youthful teenager's, known as a "face with the luster of jade." He walked down the road as though floating—graceful and light. His final immortal trans-formation was so unbelievable that it has been praised through the ages. When he was about to pass away, he said very clearly to his disciples: "Already there are many celestial beings beckoning me. I'm afraid I must leave soon." When he finally passed on, everyone watched as he "shed" his body like a cicada. Ultimately, his disci-ples were left with just a pile of clothes for a burial, and set them aside as a memorial for future generations to pay homage.

As one of the highly achieved Daoist masters I admire the most, I have read much of Sima Chengzhen's biography, life, and history. My admiration rests on his advocacy of "maintaining the ultimate emptiness" until one reaches the point where "all things become one, and one returns to emptiness." This has been my pursuit since I first turned toward the Dao. In a line, the Dao is rooted in "no mind," forgetting all emotions and attachments, purity and stillness, and non-action. Non-action is the most wondrous of all practices in Daoism. Regardless of whether it is sitting medita-tion or forming the pill, these practices all start from the concept of purity and stillness. It takes great effort and time to meditate until "not a single speck of dust settles" and not a single unclean thought arises.

Students always ask me: "I have been practicing meditation for a long time. Why have I not achieved the state spoken of in the Daoist classics?"

I reply: "Before studying meditation, I gave you several funda-mental rules. Have you come to the point in your sitting where you no longer distinguish right or wrong, good or evil? Where there is no self, no other, no time, no space, no perception and what is perceived? No methods and no Way? Moreover, no thought of 'I who am sitting in meditation?' Have you trained your meditation so thoroughly? If not, then is there a point to discussing essence, *qi*, and spirit, or the 36 methods of *daoyin*, or the 24 tips on how to reverse the *dan*? Meditation too is a matter of faith and understanding, as well as trust, but most importantly faith and confidence. Without it, you can exhaust yourself sitting all day, and certainly never enter the right state. Perseverance and willpower are crucial to continuing a meditation practice. Like blades of grass, there are many who practice meditation, yet few who achieve. Why? They are unable to persist in their effort."

The fundamental principle of Daoist inner alchemy is completely intention-free. If you have intention, sentiment, or desire, how can you enter into nothingness? If someone can meditate to the point of forgetting themselves forgetting others, forgetting their passions, forgetting the universe entirely, they have already surpassed the practice of the "three treasures" and gone into the primordial realm. This is the realm of the true immortal, but it is so very difficult to get there! Why? Old habits are difficult to break, and the force of our accustomed behavior is difficult to shift. Having already tasted the sweetness of life's pleasures, we are not able to give them up on our own. How can we be expected to sit in meditation until we wear out the mat? Only when you are capable of foregoing and not getting trapped in the idea of emptiness, even as you reach it, will you be genuinely meditating.

I remember those days when I was diligent in meditation. I explored a variety of methods. Perhaps it was my youth, but I wanted to find the quickest way to complete the path. I asked a Daoist abbot who regularly came to visit *sifu* about methods to expedite my progress in the Way. Thinking about it now, this elder abbot was kind to give me the answer he did, telling me something that, at that age, I would not have been able to fully grasp, but that would ripen with time. He said: "When you reach the point where you can grasp the pith instruction on nothingness and existence, on emptiness and being, then you're not far off!" After 1,000 searches and endless inquiries, not unlike the ancients who walked until their shoes fell apart, I also sought out all the learned scholars of the time, both north and south. All the while I held steadfast to my understanding of the phrase "Spiritual investigation must be honest, spiritual practice must be acted." This spirit of practice is of great importance to the young Daoists of the modern age who practice meditation. If you want me to speak sincerely about why afterwards I did not persist in working at sitting, perhaps it just comes from my closeness to those who were my seniors already making it clear that meditation is only a fundamental beginning, and that when you have realized why you should sit, you must then put down the mat. Letting go without a single word. You have already entered into another realm. The words appear to be in the ear, but the ancestors have already ridden the crane and vanished.

CHAPTER 44

Refining the Mind to the Miraculous Dao, Both the Person and the Way Vanish

Ever since I applied meditation to my everyday activities, walking, abiding, sitting, lying down, talking or even in silence, I gradually realized what the concepts of "not a single thought" and "the mind resides in every single object" really mean, and then moved one step further and understood this Chan poem:[1]

When the monkey is put in its place,
The elegant six windows open.
No distinction between inside and out,
No hindrance between West and East.
Greed in the heart is like fire,
Over time the hair resembles puffs of smoke.
No problems between good and bad,
Just arisings from the original emptiness.
Loosen ties to the house and boat,
The windows open together.
Smoke and mist or up and down,
Sun and moon arising from one's West and East.
Cast hasty impressions to the flowing water,
The fleeting lights are like morphing puffs of smoke.

---

1   The equivocal and abstruse nature of some literary works such as these render adequate translations nearly impossible. We have provided a translation merely for the sake of completeness, aware that it does not do justice to the original poem in Chinese.

Quietly observe every manifestation of nature,
Let the clouds purify perception of emptiness.

Later on, during my study of Chan, I realized that if it's possible to "be free from the four notions[2] and all conceptual falsehood," to be free from all dualistic thinking, to reach the stage when thoughts extinguish as they arise, when phenomena die as they come into being, to see all worldly manifestations as though watching a play, handling them with ease and utterly unfettered, then where is there such a thing as a meditation cushion, rotating the river chariot or Daoist fasting and visualization methods? All of the eight worldly concerns should be treated as in this *gatha*:[3]

Riding the waves of the play of Fate, playing around with the
king of lions,
Having been through the six dusts and out the six windows,
The lively waters conceal a dragon not yet sacrificed,
At ease across and over in the manner of Patriarchs.

To my surprise, I felt a sense of ease and tranquility, complete limpidity, and silent illumination take over me.

During those times, I heard from several elders of the Daoist school that the pithiest instruction the School of Complete Reality passed on could be summarized by the characters *qu wu*.[4] Comprehending this could lead to achieving the Way—the total realization of emptiness. As I grew older, I cumulatively compiled scores of historical materials on the interconnection of the three doctrines, namely Daoism, Confucianism, and Buddhism. According to historical resources, many School of Complete Reality patriarchs such as Wang Chongyang and Lu Dongbin, as well as the Seven Masters of the School of Complete Reality, have been quoted as articulating the sameness of Dao and Zen; from the Han to the Tang

---

2   四相 (*sixiang*): The notions of a self, an object, a sentient being, or a life span.
3   A Sanskrit word meaning "verse," "song," "stanza." A lot of Buddhist scriptures were written in *gatha* form.
4   去無. Literally, "getting rid of" and "emptiness." Unsurprisingly, the true meaning of these two seemingly simple characters, together in this context, escapes us.

and Song dynasties, many Daoist writings more or less blended Zen and Hindu philosophies. From then on, writings pertaining to breathing and transformation of the physical body arrived in rapid succession. The discourses of [Daoist] patriarchs such as Wu Chongxu easily demonstrate Confucian and Buddhist influence.

By way of further illustration, Southern School thought is largely related to Hinduism with the slight change of how *qi* travels through the pathways. Therefore, having read and consulted much historical material, I gradually came to understand what a lot of past Daoist practitioners had taught—that is, when it comes to pure Daoist alchemist practices, Wei Boyang's *Cantong Qi* provides the most reliable source of information, although it has really put later scholars to the test as those without an astonishing breadth of learning can find it extremely hard to grasp its depth. This book, together with Zhang Ziyang's *Wuzhen Pian*, will put all other [Daoist] classics to shame. If you are able to read just a few chapters of *Cantong Qi* a day, you will grow to appreciate its beautiful language which welds together scores of essential tips; and even if you can't fully understand the true meaning behind the encrypted text immediately, you will nevertheless spontaneously get a sense of blessing power by reading it this way.

An anonymous Zen poem goes like this:

Meditating over burning incense in Nantai...
Nothing troubles my mind throughout the day
It is not that I forcibly cease any thoughts from arising
For originally there is nothing there to discuss

The very last verse of this stanza in particular truly clinches the point. For quite a while, from my teens to midlife, I've heard about, as well as encountered, countless practitioners sharing what they had learned, yet hardly any of them could truly relinquish their attachment to the meditation method. In the early 1970s, I accompanied a fellow practitioner, surnamed Wu, who claimed to be possessed by demons, to visit a Daoist elder surnamed Lin at his temple. I was astonished and intrigued by a Daoist poem carved onto a plank of wood in a seal script calligraphic style.

> The way is not far, it's within you. Even though things are in essence emptiness, they are not the eternal absolute. When things are not the eternal absolute, then *qi* gets caught there. When *qi* returns to the ocean of the original eternal, then life is limitless. When the body is swamped with desire, the spirit is not free. Do not let objects of desire become caught in the spirit. When objects of desire inhabit the body, the spirit will not be clear, true essence will dissipate while strength and vitality decrease. If the spirit guards the *qi*, and the *qi* stays in the body, then there's no need to learn or practice a variety of complex methods, for you will very naturally achieve great longevity. Even though the path of practice is simple, realization is rare. And even if blessed with some realization, not all practitioners focus and persevere, so even if vast numbers of people learn, often not even one or two will truly achieve. If the spirit is free but kept in, or returned to, the body, then original *qi* will flow freely. If you maintain this day after day and night after night, then the original state of a newborn will be achieved.

Having observed Wu, Elder Lin chatted with him for a little while. First, Elder Lin reassured Wu that he hadn't gone astray, for Wu was still able to articulate his bodily sensation and his thinking remained clear. The diagnosis was that the issue arose from Wu's addiction to Chan practice. The advice was that if he could let go of his attachment to meditation by refraining from doing it for a short while, he would gradually recover. He should also avoid randomly trying just anything out of desperation. Instead, he should temporarily forget about his daily practice and use the time to engage in leisure activities and other pursuits that would relax him. Upon leaving the temple, the words of Elder Lin resonated with me. I felt as if I had just returned from a worthwhile trip, illuminated with profound insight. Elder Lin's practice path primarily follows a doctrine that teaches the essential thoughts and classics of Laozi and Zhuangzi, which all of his students are requested to study. I was deeply impressed by how he masterfully combined the theories with his own practice and applied this to his day-to-day life.

He taught that if one was able to [do something] during one's meditation, one's mind would eventually settle into tranquility on its own. This experience of tranquility can be gradually elevated to a next-level state that is void of mental effort. By then, the state [expressed in the *Dao De Jing*] of ultimate emptiness and quietude would naturally arrive, which is in line with the true meaning [of meditation]. Failing to be completely void of mental obscurations in their meditation practice, practitioners would not be able to arrive at their self-awakening nature. They would, instead, be perpetually conditioned in the relative state of subject and object. If practitioners can truly let go, a state of purity and truth can be achieved. [As in *The Book of Odes*] in the Supreme Heaven, there are no sounds or smells; it is "perfect." In Daoism, this is the idea that the original state is emptiness. By mastering the pithy instruction of the original state, practitioners can then move ahead on their path to obtain the golden elixir. Elder Lin also said that according to his own experiences, those who can truly master the pivot of meditation are at the opportune moment to achieve the state [depicted in the *Dao De Jing*] where one lightly fuses one's vital energy and returns to the gentle state [of a baby]. At this moment, the person's body will be as soft as if they have not a single bone, their fingers can be bent backwards, they will act like they are intoxicated by something, their body and mind are seemingly in a state of haziness. Elder Lin went on and told Wu that if he achieved this he would be welcome to visit him for more guidance.

In fact, whether from personal experiences or reading commentaries by past sages, I deeply and fully realized that true Dao exists between Heaven and Earth. In other words, it can be picked up just about anywhere. The key is to first enter the "transformation" stage, which unfortunately is rather mysterious and requires a capacity to understand tacitly since it cannot be described with words. All in all, if a person is able to enter the aforementioned stage while achieving what is described in the *Diamond Sutra*—to forgo the notions of a self, a person, a sentient being, and a life span—their practice will be elevated one level higher. Metaphysical speculation is still conditioned by the three planes of existence. Everything under such scope is nothing but names. Those who wish to move forward with their meditation and spiritual practices can only do so if their chosen path involves training of the mind. It is essential to note that meditating without paying attention to the mind leads to a muddled head.

If a practitioner meditates until all conditions, things, and afflictions are forgotten, they are able to drive their *qi* with their spirit; their *qi* can calm their breath, which will naturally lead to the understanding of returning to the gentlest state [of a baby]. As time passes, by continuing to maintain and nourish this gentle state without much mental force, practitioners will achieve what past Daoist immortals expressed as being at ease on all occasions; this is the ultimate level of all endeavors. Nothing external can enter nor can anything from within leak out, since at this stage there is nothing to guard nor to release. The mind is encompassing both real and not real while melding into the void until comprehension of Dao is completed.

CHAPTER 45

MASTER WENSHI— PURITY, TRANQUILITY, AND NON-ACTION

In my younger years, when I had just begun studying meditation, *sifu* gave me a stitch-bound book entitled *The Perfect Classic of the Beginning of the Scripture of the Supreme Way*.[1] He said the work was included in the *Complete Library in Four Sections*.[2] The lettering of this copy was crisp and beautiful. Even though I didn't yet understand most of the content, I read it with enormous delight. *Sifu* encouraged me to read it aloud as one would chant a sutra, saying that over time the meaning would become clear to me.

The Daoist master Guan Yinzi is the author of this book. A contemporary of Laozi, he was originally a senior official in the Zhou Dynasty. Later, during the rule of King Zhao of Zhou, he was appointed to serve as chief magistrate of Hangu Pass. This was a low-maintenance post, in which he was responsible for customs inspections and generally overseeing the traffic of goods through the area.

Since childhood, Guan Yinzi had been fascinated with the *Yi Jing* and the *Su Shu*[3] as well as astronomy and geography. Through his own research, he had learned much about these subjects. He took advantage of his relaxed professional life at Hangu Pass to

---

1 無上妙道文始真經 (*wu shang miao dao wen shi zhen jing*).
2 四庫全書 (*siku quanshu*): The largest encyclopedic collection of books in Chinese history, compiled during the Qing dynasty upon orders from the Qianlong Emperor, it contained over 10,000 titles, and compendiums of over 4,000. Also known as the *Imperial Collection of Four Divisions* or the *Complete Library of Four Branches of Books*.
3 素書: A guide on how to live in the world ethically, said to have been written by Zhang Liang (張良) during the Western Han Dynasty (3rd century BCE).

progress [in his thirst for knowledge], reading all the great works available. He had long admired Laozi's writings on ethics as well as his practical demonstration of the principles. One day, Laozi, riding on an ox, happened to make his way through Hangu Pass. When Guan Yinzi heard the news, he was overjoyed. He went to the gate to greet the master and ensure he was received with ample hospitality. Upon meeting Laozi, Guan Yinzi began to kowtow, intending to demonstrate the highest degree of reverence possible, but Laozi firmly refused to let him perform these gestures. Guan Yinzi remained determined and sometime later went to meet Laozi again to ask for guidance in Daoist practice. He also appealed to the master to compile his teachings into a book that could be passed down to later generations.

Guan Yinzi continued to treat Laozi with the utmost respect, attending to him as a disciple would a master and humbly requesting guidance on questions. Thus, after silently observing Guan Yinzi for a period of time, Laozi agreed [to teach him]. Guan Yinzi immediately resigned from his official post and began traveling with Laozi as the master spread the wisdom of the Dao throughout the land. They eventually reached Boyang, Guan Yinzi's hometown, and decided to settle in the auspicious area of Longshan. There, they received visitors who had a karmic connection and guided them in pursuit of the Dao. Over their many years together, Laozi used every spare moment to share all that he had studied and realized over his lifetime. [Later], Laozi recorded the essence of his life's insights in a book, the *Dao De Jing*. He entrusted the book to Guan Yinzi and told him to study it with utmost care. Laozi advised his disciple that whatever epiphanies he had, he should not forget that wisdom arises from the Dao and should be shared with all sentient beings who are fated to understand. Laozi then set off to travel on his own again. Guan Yinzi's life was imbued with its own karmic destiny. His mystical connection to the ancient canon had motivated him to study the texts diligently since childhood. After receiving guidance from Laozi, his learning and practice progressed rapidly. His comprehension deepened further after additional years of pouring over the *Dao De Jing*. Subsequently, he expanded upon the teachings of the *Dao De Jing* in the *Wen Shi Zhen Jing* [*The Perfect Classic of the Beginning of the Scripture of the Supreme Way*]. In total, the work comprises nine sections.

In the classes that I attended back when I was studying at *sifu*'s residence, *sifu* was constantly bringing up these works by Guan Yinzi. He spoke about the key ideas of the book's nine sections at every opportunity in his lectures. *Sifu* did not merely admire Guan Yinzi for his practice and his writings; he also revered the ancient master's humility and the self-restraint that he maintained through pure emptiness. Zhuangzi, who came after Guan Yinzi, also held Guan Yinzi in high regard, and later generations of Daoist practitioners have all referred to Guan Yinzi as "the supreme spiritual master." Before Guan Yinzi even met Laozi, he was already well known as a scholar. Even the Zhou Dynasty ruler admired Guan Yinzi's character and erudition, and was intrigued by the mysterious lore that followed him. Thus, the ruler conferred upon him the great honor of a senior official rank. But Guan Yinzi's whole mind was set on the way of the Dao, so he had no ambition for fame or profit. He attempted to resign from his official position many times without success. Finally, he was appointed to the lowly position of managing traffic through Hangu Pass, during which time he was able to spend more time studying the sacred texts. According to *sifu*, the ancient masters [like Guan Yinzi] devoted themselves to the Dao with a determination that has been unmatched in later generations of practitioners. Guan Yinzi used his expertise in astronomy to study the stars. After he ascertained from the sky that a noble person would soon come through Hangu Pass, he thoroughly cleaned his home, and he bathed and fasted every day leading up to the arrival. He went about all these preparations in the hope that he would have a chance for an audience with the holy guest. He wished to request guidance in the Dao. *Sifu* described these events in vivid and moving detail. Ultimately, Laozi looked upon Guan Yinzi with the full force of his saintly insight and perceived the depth of his respect. Laozi also recognized Guan Yinzi's ability and potential as a Daoist practitioner. Such talented disciples were uncommon, and so Laozi gladly accepted him. Thereafter, the old master transmitted to Guan Yinzi his whole life's worth of profound insight.

Sifu commented that those who have come after Guan Yinzi have no way to fully comprehend the wisdom in his writings. Therefore, *sifu* instructed that seekers could only begin from meditation. It is essential that they only receive the teachings that their karmic connection allows.

This is some of what *sifu* shared with me regarding the *Wen Shi Zhen Jing*. On a particular day of teaching on this text, he made a special point to share a story from his youth: when he was seeking the Dao at Huashan, his karmic destiny guided him to receive oral tips from both the Huashan and Louguan Schools. *Sifu* said that now most people speak of the Wen Shi School, but the esteemed ancestors of Daoism used the term "*Louguan*" for these teachings. *Sifu* also advised using any free time for additional study of the *Kai Tian Jing* and the *Miao Zhen Jing*.[4] He then traced the entire lineage of the Daoist school of which he had been speaking, from the Wei, Jin, and Northern and Southern Dynasties all the way to the Tang and Song period. He named each famous Daoist elder in this history as well as the achievements and events of every age. Once he reached the Tang Dynasty, he listed all of the Daoist priests and told the anecdotes associated with each of them.

Students of the *Wen Shi Zhen Jing* who have applied themselves to it for some time, reading it over and over, may gradually come to understand the teaching that Zhuangzi quoted in his own writing. This is the main point of Guan Yinzi's work:

> To the person that does not dwell in themselves, the form of things shows itself just as it is. This person's movements are like water, stillness like a mirror and responses like echoes. They are so transparent, it is as if they have disappeared, their solidarity is in clearness, with others they are harmonious, and they see

---

4   開天經, 妙真經: The *Scripture on the Opening of the Heavens* and *Sublime Scripture*, two early Daoist classics, dealing with cosmology.

gains as losses. Rather than taking precedence over others, they follow them.

This passage is from the third section of the *Wen Shi Zhen Jing*. It explains how to relinquish attachments to meaningless appearances and offers a complete revelation of the realm of true emptiness. The text also expounds upon the essential concepts of non-dual awareness and the oneness of meditation and wisdom.

The teachings are powerful, as if to shock people awake. The text instructs seekers to release all attachments, and it reveals the state of cohesion achieved by those extraordinary practitioners who have entered the holy realm. They understand the non-differentiation between movement and stillness and are completely at ease, without hindrance. Flowing like water, as limpid as a mirror, the full intentions of their hearts are manifested without hindrance, and the secular world becomes like a game unfolding within their state of intense meditation.

After reading this text, I became convinced of Guan Yinzi's wisdom. In fact, the realm he describes is the same as the *Prajna* consciousness spoken of by the Buddhists. It's not surprising that Zhuangzi, almost 100 years after Guan Yinzi, regarded him as a spiritual master of exceedingly lofty stature. Accordingly, Zhuangzi enthusiastically devoted himself to the master's teachings and promoted them tirelessly to later generations.

In any case, Guan Yinzi's legacy from his manifestation in the material world is extensive. His teachings call for people to purify their internal landscape and rely on tranquility. Outwardly, seekers must act with modesty and self-reliance, in the manner of a gentleman.

He also advocated caution in words and actions, and abandonment of contrived efforts so that all [that is fated/that is to be done] can be manifested instead through natural non-action. [Moreover, the text instructs that] whether in the spiritual realm or in dealing with the outside world, people cannot force their way. The [ideal] is to flow like water, moving organically, never obstructed but never acting aggressively or in pursuit of some contrived end.

The practitioner's way in the Dao is free from artifice. Their mind is an expanse of emptiness, and they are not controlled by the material world or attachments. Thus, they are not afflicted with sadness. Their solitary spirit follows an independent standard, simultaneously boundless and unconstrained. And they return frequently to observe their own mind.

Guan Yinzi regularly guided followers of the Daoist way toward enlightenment, while always [abiding by the principles] of emptiness and non-action. He eschewed all worldly pursuits. Instead, he flowed through his existence like a deep, clear river. He was without attachments or pursuits; and rather than actively seeking to be the one to lead, he always followed others. In this, his great wisdom and foresight are evident. He perceived realities that were invisible to regular human beings. On one occasion, Liezi asked Guan Yinzi: "How is it that those who have achieved the Dao can be immersed in water but not drown, enter flames but not burn, and walk along overhanging cliffs with complete ease, not a trace of fear in their mind nor a tremor of anxiety in their body? I find it all very curious. What factors underlie these phenomena?"

Guan Yinzi replied to Liezi: "Only those who have accessed the purest *yang qi* from the cosmos can [reach this state]. These feats are not the product of earthly skill or knowledge, nor of risky impulses." In sum, all of Guan Yinzi's works focus on the meaning of tranquility and non-action. From start to finish, his writings both advocate and embody these principles. Clearly Laozi's legacy was etched upon Guan Yinzi, as if the old master had been reincarnated.

CHAPTER 46

LET GO OF ALL KARMIC TIES—RETURN THE GAZE TOWARD SELF-NATURE

As I matured and got bumped and battered by the ebb and flow of life's experiences, so my view and understanding of meditation changed. In addition, after periodically revisiting *The Perfect Classic of the Beginning of the Scripture of the Supreme Way*, the *Cantong Qi*, and the *Yellow Court Classic*, I no longer got caught up in the external forms of meditation. Perhaps it is like the *gatha*: "The bodhisattva in you has never left; it has become a distant stranger in your dark house; once the meditative light reflects inwards, you'll find the ancient housemaster, there before birth." After you genuinely understand your mind's nature, you can maintain its proper upkeep in any place. No matter what phenomena you come across, direct your search inward, and each and every moment becomes meditation.

I am filled with admiration and gratitude for those who have sought the Dao in the past. Perhaps because of good karma in a past life, I have been able to meet with many teachers. They are not all necessarily famous, but I am absolutely convinced that each one of these illumined masters walked and realized the true path of pure practice for themselves. Householder Huang Dabai was one such master whom I would later visit, a practitioner of both Buddhism and Daoism and a great adept hidden in plain sight of the world. In his early years, he took refuge in both Master Taixu and Empty Cloud,[1] and studied the Dao on Qingcheng Mountain. It is

---

1   虛雲: Xu Yun, one of the greatest Chan Buddhist teachers of the 19th and 20th centuries.

said that he meditated for over 50 years. Through my interaction with him, it's clear to me that the authenticity and profundity of his explanation on the transformation of the four elements of physical form is solidly built on real experiences and is in no way a baseless fabrication blurted out without basis.

I greatly agree with his inclusion of the Śūraṅgama Sūtra[2] as an important addition to the Daoist's spiritual literature. The sutra's elucidation of the "50 demonic states" is especially crucial for a Daoist practitioner's inner examination. Many Daoist meditators will end up overly attached to the physical aspect of their training, forgetting that the most important element is still the mind. If you meditate like a rigid board, staying wrapped up in names and the sensations and perceptions that come with training the meridians and channels, your meditation will never reach the higher levels of practice.

Huang, the elder householder, once said to me that in his 90 years of life, he had studied closely with nearly all of the great masters of his age. He had received the high teachings of the four schools of Vajrayana Buddhism and gone on two retreats in mainland China just to taste the transcendent wonders of *phowa*.[3] Within the Hinayana tradition he had also practiced the "White Skeleton Meditation"[4] and witnessed the sacred light emitting from the bones. Later he had personally followed a yogi of the ancient Shaktism School, and practiced *chod*[5] many times within the charnel grounds. He said something to me that really got me thinking: contrary to his expectations, those few experiences of offering his body in the graveyard had actually intensified his body's transformational process. At the very moment he gave up

---

2 One of the most important sutras of the *Mahāyāna* Buddhist canon.

3 頗瓦法 (*powafa*): Yogic practice whereby the practitioner learns to "eject" consciousness from the body with the aim of directing it after death. Higher-level practitioners can also assist the transmigration of the consciousness of others after death.

4 白骨觀 (*baiguguan*): Meditative practice whereby the practitioner meditates on the decomposition of a corpse from death to dust. One major benefit is the reduction of desire.

5 施身法 (*shishenfa*): Yogic practice where the practitioner offers his body to spirits.

the existence of his body, he accomplished the complete opening of his eight extraordinary channels and the conception and governing vessels. In the midst of his practice, he managed to completely shatter all notions of, and clinging to, a "body," whereupon he was able to see how a single-minded obsession with perceptions of an independently existing self actually becomes an obstruction to the pursuit of the Way.

He went on to say that Buddhism has its unique and unmatched aspects. If a Daoist practitioner is able to let go of all perceptions of the existence of a "body" that they cling to during the process, using non-action as their principal method and applying "no mind" throughout, they will arrive at the state where "not a single thought arises." Of importance is how one can enter the genuine state where not a single thought arises. Through the lens of Buddhism, this state predicates thoroughly letting go of the mind and body, the channels and meridians of *qi*, bright spots, and such things as an elixir or acupoints. Abandoning these, you will naturally step closer to accomplishing the non-arising state. Without the elements of *Prajna* and emptiness in your meditation, you cannot hope to reach greater heights in your practice.

Yongzheng, in his early years as an emperor during the Qing Dynasty, carried a deep bitterness in his alchemical training. Under the influence of his over-affection for the Daoist elixir, he could see no way through. Only later, when devoting himself to Chan practice, could he see faintly that another path had revealed itself. Exasperated, he told Zhang Jia, the national teacher to the emperor and a Buddhist master in his own right, about his experience of enlightenment during his Chan practice. Zhang Jia concluded frankly that his enlightenment was just the shadow and sliver of it, and that Yongzheng had not penetrated deeply enough. Yongzheng then knew that the only way for him to walk the true Way was to let go of all bodily perception and attachment.

It is just like what is said in the Śūraṅgama Sūtra: on the plane of existence, with all of its mountains, rivers, and everything between, there is not one thing that isn't the creation of your wondrous, unfathomable true mind. Knowing this, there is absolutely no need to be attached to anything. Even if you were instructed to sit, since there's no one sitting, no object of meditation, and no method, you still wouldn't reach the peak. In truth, if any desire or expectation creeps into your meditation, it is frivolous. The great path does not and has never departed from your mind. Our troubles are rooted in our practiced iron grip; as we strengthen our hold on the things we care about, so do those things make us chase ever harder, ever further, leaving behind our pure, clear mind the minute the pursuit begins. What are you to do about this? You must give up everything: give up chasing your thoughts, even give up your pure and tranquil mind. If all of your channels were blocked before, they will naturally open. Do you believe it? You will know when you go there yourself.

As I meditated through the years, I put a good deal of effort into researching the array of Daoist terminology coined, created, and passed down through generations of patriarchs, Daoist immortals, and elder practitioners. These colorful locutions serve many functions: to distinguish and pinpoint, and to ensure that students don't mistake one thing for the other when being instructed by the teacher. Each school has their own set of "heirlooms," unique codes whose underlying meaning and directions can only be recognized among the schools' members. In the present day, with the whirl of information available through science and cloud technology, it would be misguided to fall prey to this same pattern of old, hoarding ancient terms and names like collector's items, and refusing to assimilate today's multifarious viewpoints and findings from scientific research. If today's practitioners go about their studies in this way, there will be little benefit for later generations. When the time comes, these warehouses of books and classics will meet the tragic end of becoming nothing more than saved files on a computer disk, with no one interested in actually studying them.

All of the Daoist wisdom of old breeds virtue and goodness wherever it is spread. It is the bloodline of the sages, meant, like all religions, to be infused seamlessly into the daily lives of every generation. Protection and care of each generation's body, mind, and spirit has always been its aim, and we can already see how Daoism and its adherents are rising to the occasion to contribute to this generation's new ideas of physical and mental health. Is it unfortunate, then, that from the Qing Dynasty, in order to prevent secret teachings from being revealed to the world, many "decoys" were created? This had led to the teachings dying out, and the truth lying amongst many mutated versions of it.

As for the 50 demonic states mentioned in the Śūraṅgama Sūtra, in the beginning of the sutra the Buddha explains the need to return one's observation to one's self-nature during any spiritual practice or in experiencing any internal or external state. This is the only way to avoid falling into the pit of false knowledge and false views. The works of Guan Yinzi, Laozi, and the sages of history do not waver from this same principle. Similarly, the Wen Shi School also advocates non-action as its highest principle. It refers to a free-flowing consciousness that does not contrive the actions of the awareness or the body. The profundity of it surpasses even the high-level achievement of Daoist alchemy. It does not feign to be greater than the process of refining essence into *qi*, transforming *qi* into spirit, and returning spirit into emptiness. However, if there is attachment to this process of refinement, then it becomes con-trived action. Within Daoism, all methods prescribe function to "gather" and "replenish," or to absorb energy and essence from the environment. They are there simply as "doctor's tools," so there's no need to get too wrapped up in them. Many people use the Southern School's methods for gathering and replenishing as excuses to play tricks on others, damaging their hidden virtues, thinking little about the fact that what is to be gathered is positive, pure *qi* from the world around them. Do not be fooled into anything that smells of greed or obscenity.

CHAPTER 47

No Desire, No Selfishness—
The True Mind Is
Without Hindrance

Before enlightenment on the path of meditation and the Dao, the greater part of a practitioner's efforts should be concentrated on the perceptions that arise in their consciousness. During the course of meditation training, the mind will move with delusive and differentiating forms so numerous that it will be impossible to keep clear track of them all. If anything arises during this that is "untrue" and we cannot hold onto our meditative stillness, many subtle obstacles can creep in. The Daoist phrase "straying into the fire, the demons take hold" isn't a depiction of possession by actual demons; it personifies the inner demons of one's mind. If you become carelessly attached to a particular form of practice, you may become the plaything of *yin* demons or other ghosts and spirits. For example, if a demon from the heavens took notice of you, but you hadn't developed any substantial skill in your meditation practice, then it would not be of great concern; but if you had already advanced far in your meditative stillness, perhaps inching close to enlightenment, then it would be a very different story.

Look at the lives of the Seven Masters of Complete Reality, or the Eight Immortals: not a single one was without obstacles. Why is this? Demons from the heavens are terrified of someone realizing the Dao. The second it happens, their palaces tremble and the earth quakes violently, without end. Thus, they will employ any means to waylay your progress, to coerce you into abandoning your spiritual pursuits, to bar you from reaching the final fruits of your labors.

Those who waver easily in their stillness may suffer the harassment of *chi mei*[1] spirits.

There was once an old practitioner, from the Tainan Guan Temple, who had reached a considerable level of proficiency in meditative stillness. Despite his meditative acumen, faint dreams of reputation and success occasionally slipped through his mind, luring him into mundanity. After a chance encounter with a woman, he found himself utterly incapable of calming his mind during meditation. At the root of it, his mind still held some unresolved worldly afflictions, and the demon struck at his weakness. He, like the veritable fields of fallen practitioners before him, was unable to recover.

The thing a practitioner of Daoist meditation most dreads is becoming blind with foolish affections born out of ignorance. In regard to this, I often give beginners some suggestions. The disposition of most beginner meditators is with the *yang qi* concentrated in the area of the lower *dantian*. This makes uncontrolled erections all too likely to occur. Explained in Daoist terms, as you approach the stage of gathering the small medicine, you will experience a feeling of warmth in the area between your belly button and rectum. Without proper guidance, meditators at this stage are susceptible to leakage [of seminal fluids]. Those with greater strength of mind and fewer stray thoughts, who can remain unaffected by the pull of their desires, will use this chance to deepen their commitment and pivot toward the next level of their practice.

The bliss one experiences at this stage makes the most stimulating sexual pleasure seem bland, and herein lies the problem. Daoists will know it is necessary to employ "real breathing" to gather the small medicine, and a crucial component of this breathing is related to the state of one's own mind. Not only must the mind avoid latching onto phenomena, but breathing must be regulated until it no longer happens through the nose or mouth.

---

1   魑魅: A particular kind of supernatural beings/demons from the mountains, who took on a human face and the body of a beast. They are mentioned in the Śūraṅgama Sūtra and in many classics of Chinese literature.

To go a bit further into it, if you could cut off and never give rise to another sexual thought, you would have already reached the point of having stopped all leakage. Were you surrounded by ghosts, spirits, goblins, and sprites, they would be unable to do anything to you. Why? Here's a secret: all demons exist within the realm of the greedy, desirous mind. Therefore, the transformation of desires rests with the mind, not in sitting. The day you are able to let go of your lust, desires, and attachments, is the day you will be naturally replete with essence, *qi*, and spirit. Ghosts and spirits will be unable to take advantage of you.

The Śūraṅgama Sūtra illustrates this point with precision and clarity. At that time, the Buddha said to Ananda: "Inverting the gaze toward one's self-nature, and observing until the end is reached: by this alone one can depart from all perceptions of thought and object; by this alone one gains complete clarity and stillness; through this all mental disturbances lose their power." In short, regardless of whichever method you use to practice, everything must always return to the mind. Taking into additional consideration the caliber of practitioners of the modern era, the Śūraṅgama Sūtra's 50 demonic states still stand as an essential companion and an excellent barometer in clearly discerning your own mind and checking for any signs of deviation from the path.

I had the good fortune to discover the teachings of the "three peaks" of Confucianism, Buddhism, and Daoism, while still in my late teens. I am ashamed to say that, for the decades that I have traversed this mountain range, I have done little but trip and stumble in my weakness, fiddling away the days in jest, a bag of bones empty of qualifications, and full of sighs. I have only mastered how to confuse and befuddle others. One thing I can say to console myself is something my *sifu* once said: "If you're heart's in the right place, unintentional faults in your words can be mended." It was only after a decade of persistent prodding from students and fellow practitioners that I decided two or three years ago, after long and careful deliberation, to put pen to paper and share an arbitrary smattering of my recollections in the study of the Dao. I cannot imagine how this will make for a good read, with the thousand things I've left out, and much of what is in here isn't the stuff of secret transmissions, but just sincere words I write for the sake of my own happiness. However, in light of the instructions and precepts left to me from the days under the tutelage of my *sifu*, sometimes the best I can hope for is to leave some people of this generation with general concepts of the study of Daoism, superficial as my words may be. If I have been unable to uncover the roots and explain them each in a thorough, satisfactory way, I offer my sincere apologies.

To explain meditation in a way that makes sense and won't create too much pressure for the interested beginners of today, [I would say] try to build the foundation of your meditation on the cultivation of health and virtue. Twenty years ago, I went to visit a temple in Fengshan, outside Kaohsiung. The instructors there were giving an interesting explanation on how to enter into meditative stillness. They said you must be able to forget everything. Before you sit, first you must remember to take all the personal things you can forget and completely discard them, including your body, and when you've reached this state of absolute abandonment, you are ready to sit. Our biggest attachment is the things around us that we can feel, see, touch, think about, and use. They are all hard to put down, which means we enter into meditation with all of this baggage, the source of our delusive thoughts and attachments.

To really practice meditation, you must completely let go of all things, emotions, circumstances, appearances, and desires. You must even let go of the idea of "I" and "other." If you can do this, your meditation certainly might make some progress. Gradually, you will also be able to empty your mind during meditation, empty your space, and empty your bad habits. Another impediment to meditation is the desire to go fast and achieve milestones quickly. So long as you seek to hasten your progress, you will have many obstacles. The best method for dealing with the obstacles that arise in your meditation is to discreetly accumulate good deeds and virtue, as well as to often practice making offerings. Past masters were wont to say that if you want to reach heights in your cultivation of the Dao, you must first establish yourself firmly in virtuous conduct, in the vein of Yuan Liaofan, who changed the course of his destiny through his daily accumulation of good deeds. Some scriptures even go so far as to say that all the apparent virtuous behaviors are limited in nature, whereas the merit of hidden virtuous acts is immeasurable. The highest form of offering, which yields the greatest merit, is one that is formless, whereby there is no giver, receiver, or offering made. Meditators must guard against their essence and spirit from leaking out, for which the cultivation of no mind is of paramount importance and should be cultivated until devoid of any trace of greed, anger, and ignorance, until all sense of gain and loss has gone, and all notion of auspicious, ill-boding, or disaster are done away with. Gradually, as you cultivate and guard this inner capacity, your essence, *qi*, and spirit will naturally blossom. If the mind does not scatter outward, one's essence will not leak out, one's *qi* will not dissolve out, and one's spirit will not flow out. Throughout their daily doings, meditators should strive to be away from their six roots, in a state of no mind, empty of wants and worries, and should regulate themselves and attend to others with an upright and sincere mind. Their mind should be fearless in the face of life or death because the mind that dwells on the dichotomy of life and death is the enemy to longevity. When you run into situations, deal with them unhurriedly, peacefully, and respond accordingly, and in your relationships with others strive to be humble.

Practitioners of Daoist meditation ought to use destitution as a teacher. If you are able to understand the meaning of destitution, wouldn't you be content even if you had nothing more than a bowl of rice and a glass of water for sustenance? In any situation, at any time, in any place, keep an attitude of going beyond the mundane, with the ease and freedom of someone who is both beyond the world but in it, or never leaving it but being beyond it. Regardless of whether sitting or in motion, discrimination in thought or method can never arise during meditation. Especially avoid attachment to words, to language, to expression. The fear is that stasis of the mind will result from holding to any form, to any "way."

You must sit until the theory and practice are unobstructed; sit until no forms remain; sit until you see your original nature and then let go even of your original nature; sit until you can no longer sit. This is the foundation. Then, sit until there are no appearances, no mountains, rivers, or earth, and even the wondrously luminous true mind is forgotten. This is the state of deep, clear stillness, where dream and waking reality meld as one. This is called the eye that does not sleep, and it sees clearly through all dreams. If the mind abides in suchness, all phenomena are contained in one. This is the high road of meditation.

CHAPTER 48

EXCEEDING THE WORLD, THE ORDINARY IS THE DAO

I appreciate Liezi much more than Zhuangzi, perhaps owing to the fact that while Zhuangzi advocated metaphysics, Liezi was this mysterious character espousing the concept of non-intention and non-action. Liezi once followed the incredible Master Huzi, a very famous Daoist thinker and philosopher during the Warring States period. One could say he was one of the most important representatives following after Laozi. Very few of his writings exist in the world: only a few remain from the question and answer sessions between him and his disciples. Nonetheless, after studying the Dao with Huzi for nine years, Liezi had learned how to fly freely. Books tell the tale of how he could ride the winds of the Eight Directions—that is, once his intention to fly arose, he could soar above the world, flying in any direction. He most frequently rode the winds around springtime, and although the places he passed by were barren farming areas, they somehow would suddenly revive and flourish, much like after the spring rains. It is no wonder, then, that among all the Chinese rulers who upheld Daoism through the following generations, there wasn't a single one who didn't confer a high and lofty honorific title to him, including Immortal Perfect Emptiness and True Lord of Perfect Emptiness and Stillness.

In terms of the study of ethics, both Liezi's moral character and his doctrines were highly revered by scholars of later generations. Everyone considered Liezi's Daoist thought and doctrine to never deviate from the basic concept of "non-action." The way he treated others and conducted himself was also fully in line with the standards of the ancient "Six Classics." Liezi emphasized emptiness, meaning that when practicing Daoism, one must first expel all delusive thoughts from one's mind. Don't let these delusive thoughts damage and influence your original nature of peaceful non-action! One must aspire to practice until one is no longer attached to one's body and mind, nor to the notion of self and others, honor and disgrace; until one becomes one with the world, as natural and innocent as a newborn, surpassing all the thoughts, confusions, and distinctions between gain and loss in the human realm. As to the supreme state that Liezi advocated for and pursued his whole life, the so-called state of immortals, of realized beings, of the transformed ones, one ought to practice until one has become united with the natural world, with no differentiation between life and death, right and wrong, or even day and night. Only then can such aforementioned honors be bestowed upon the practitioner. Liezi's wisdom indeed surpassed that of all the great Daoist figures of later generations, even that of all Western science of today. Millennia ago, he already clearly understood the path and orbits of the planets and stars in the cosmos—indeed, early on in his books, he was already espousing such views as heliocentrism and the limitless nature of the universe.

Regarding how Liezi began to study the Dao from his master, he was full of curiosity, much like we are in the modern age. At that time, there was a very famous shaman named Ji Xian, who was expert at knowing other's good and bad fortune, particularly the date and time of one's death. His predictions were very rarely not spot on and he was quite revered by the locals. One day, upon another's recommendation, Liezi sought Ji Xian, asking for insight into his future through divination. Who would have thought that Liezi was so spellbound by the shaman's words that he prostrated himself before him, going so far as to think that Ji Xian's skills surpassed even those of his teacher Huzi! Upon returning to his master's dwelling, then, he said to him: "Until today, I always thought that *sifu*'s Daoist methods were the greatest under heaven. Now I know that there is one who is even greater than *sifu*!"

Huzi listened, without any reaction or expression. He simply gently replied to his disciple: "You have studied here with me for a bit, and at the moment all you've gained is a little trick, a half-baked understanding of the techniques. And now you want to go and study with someone ever higher! The other's experience far surpasses yours, so you would naturally be deceived. If you don't believe me, have him come here and tell my fortune!"

Hence, Liezi brought Ji Xian to Huzi's residence on many occasions, yet every time, the student was tricked by the teacher. The first time, the master appeared to be about to die, fooling Liezi into crying uncontrollably. The next time, *sifu* appeared to be rising from the dead, being reborn full of vitality. This made even Ji Xian stare, dumbfounded. The third time, Huzi appeared to be in a dispirited and depressed mental state, making Ji Xian unable to properly tell his fortune. Finally, the fourth time, Huzi thought the right opportunity had arrived, and he appeared to the shaman as he truly was. And who would have thought it! As Liezi led Ji Xian to his teacher's quarters, upon entering the shaman turned around and ran away so quickly, his feet hadn't even stepped onto the floor of the house! Huzi told Liezi to bring Ji Xian back. The student chased after him for quite a while, only to return to his teacher's home to say that the shaman had already disappeared, leaving no trace, making it impossible for him to keep up. Then, Liezi humbly bowed and respectfully asked Huzi: "What exactly has been going on, from beginning to end?"

Huzi casually replied, as if playing it down: "I just showed him formlessness, something that someone with his capacity simply cannot fathom. Thus, he revealed himself for what he truly is! Had he not run away, could it be that he would have humiliated himself?"

After this incident, aside from feeling a deep sense of guilt toward his master, and repenting profusely, Liezi also came to a sudden realization. For the following three years, he shut himself away at home, performing household chores such as cooking, doing laundry, and feeding the livestock. In addition, he began interacting with people and treating others in a much more natural way than before. He maintained a simple kind of manner, free of desires and overthinking, keeping a distance from all worldly affairs. Once, this used to be the kind of life I envied and yearned for, because it was ultimately just like the final state described in Chan Buddhism—seeing the mountain as mountain, seeing the water as water. From then on, I thought the way of practice should at the very minimum be like that of Liezi: unfettered, utterly at ease living or dying, surpassing the achievement of Daoist immortals, a state to which possessing transformative powers cannot even be compared.

Later generations of Daoist scholars were deeply influenced by Liezi. Yet, most go through piles and piles of Daoist texts—enough to fill a house to the rafters—but rarely can they genuinely grasp their essence. After comprehending the Dao, for 40 years Liezi lived a carefree, quiet life in seclusion in the state of Zheng, a life more ordinary than that of any ordinary person, in which he rejected all court requests and titles. Had he not already unfettered himself from all the eight worldly affairs, how could he be content with the way things were? During these 40 years, Liezi compiled the essence of his life's studies into 20 volumes consisting of over 100,000 characters. But these volumes suffered as a result of the chaos of war. Although later scholars tried to preserve and collect them, the complete version had been lost, and only about eight volumes remain. Later generations were left stumbling around in the dark, some putting emphasis on the mythological aspects of Liezi's writings, which is truly a pity. People rarely investigate the reason why such an incredible person was able to live for a full 40 years in the state of Zheng, completely unnoticed even by his next-door neighbors! Could it be possible he had already practiced to the state that Laozi had described as "softening the glare and unifying with the mundane"?

CHAPTER 49

Referring to the *Cantong Qi*, One Begins to Comprehend Their Roots

If I were to speak frankly, since the times of Laozi and Liezi, Wei Boyang from the Eastern Han Dynasty is someone I truly respect. Ge Hong only described him in a few simple sentences, saying that he was born from nobility, being fond of the way of the Dao his whole life. He was never interested in official positions in bureaucracy, throughout his whole life emphasizing moral and spiritual character. He concealed his identity, and to the people of his day he was a hermit shrouded in mystery. Fervently focused on the study of the Daoist canon, he devoted his entire life to writing, and was thus able to produce a Daoist tome incomparable to anything at the time: the *Cantong Qi*. This work has left a powerful, lasting influence over the generations. When it came into the world, everyone revered it as a precious treasure, yet its contents were so enormous and profound that it was hard to fathom. In the centuries since, who knows how many distinguished Daoist sages have immersed themselves in this book, unable to draw a definite conclusion, or even comprehend its main threads! No wonder that many of those who wrote commentaries and annotations to it did so under an alias, careful not to damage the literary fame they had built up their whole lives!

Had Chinese Daoist culture not had Wei's *Cantong Qi* as a pillar for the past millennia, its splendor and magnificence surely would have been diminished. Comprehending the principles of the *Cantong Qi* is equivalent to understanding the trajectory of the movement of both the outer macrocosm of the universe and the inner microcosm within the body. It covers how the *qian* (Heaven) and *kun* (Earth) hexagrams in the *Yi Jing* are used as a portal for the coming and going of *yin* and *yang*. In addition, it explains why *wuji* (unboundedness) is in the state of true emptiness, as well as why Heaven and Earth arise from *taiji* (the absolute). The differentiation between *yin* and *yang*, leading finally to the 64 hexagrams that can be used to derive all the things and being of the universe, along with all the changes between fortune and disaster, can all be said to arise from the original hexagrams *qian* and *kun*. And from these two hexagrams extend the 64 hexagrams, inferring the good and bad fortune of the entire world, societies, families, and individuals. The application of the eight trigrams to the organs of the body is a later development of the system.

The point of Daoist practice is to use the human body to return to the inborn, innate state. This requires practicing until the ordinary body transforms and forms the golden pill, subsequently signifying "immortality." The laws of the trajectory of the eight trigrams, other than conforming to the assemblage of the River Diagram and Luo Shu Square to apply to astronomy and the creation of calendars, are also the base for the formation of water and air within the natural world. In fact, they are inseparable from the five elements—namely metal, wood, water, fire, and earth—along with the principle of the "Six Breaths."[1] To build a foundation of Daoist meditation, one must rely on the principle of returning back to its original, innate, inborn state—all that which within life's microcosm has been misplaced, lost, or turned upside-down. This is the goal of practice. Moreover, why does every month have 30 days? Why does every year have 12 months? Why must we differentiate the course of one year into 24 solar terms? This has all accordingly assembled and come about on the basis of *yin* and *yang* and the ten

---

1   六氣 (*liuqi*): The breaths of nature, of Heaven, namely: wind (風 *feng*), cold (寒 *han*), summer heat (暑 *shu*) or heat (熱 *re*), humidity (濕 *shi*), drought (燥 *zao*), and fire (火 *huo*). Their interplay gives rise to all conditions and affects the functioning of the internal organ systems of the body, causing all kinds of malaises.

heavenly stems and the 12 earthly branches. The scriptures used basic math of the ten heavenly stems and 12 earthly stems to create the perfect number of 64 hexagrams.

The profundity of the *Cantong Qi* can be found in how its intrinsic order can be applied to practices related to the physical form. Even the basic principle of the five elements can be used as a standard for cultivation. How does the waxing and waning of the moon correspond with the success of meditation and concocting the pill, along with how to control the strength and speed in the crucial moment? Within the 12 two-hour periods of the day, how is breath divided into *yin* and *yang*? Even in terms of the times of the year, different practices are applied during their corresponding seasons. [In the book] the ebb and flow of *yin* and *yang*, as well as its process, all have thorough explanations, from laying the foundations to the conception and nourishing stages—in the ten years it takes to fully develop the golden elixir, nothing can be reversed, no mistake remedied.

Not only that, but the book also mentions how to transform the 84,000 delusions and afflictions which manifest from the seven emotions and six desires. The six roots are purified and one is without intention; one meditates until the six roots no longer cling to external stimuli. In short, if one is able to encounter a wise and experienced master and thoroughly understand the content of the *Cantong Qi*, it is akin to holding the precious jewel from under the legendary black dragon's chin, at which point immortality is not far away. Wei Boyang was fully aware that it is challenging to accurately grasp the subtlety of one's essence, *qi*, and spirit in the process of meditation to create the pill. As a result, he came up with the hexagram form, and applied it to Daoist practitioners so that they know when to retreat or advance and appropriately control timing and temperature. Thus, correctly practicing in accordance with the River Diagram and Luo Shu Square to take in the *yin* and *yang* to be commanded under the *qian* and *kun* trigrams, as long as one receives directions from a wise master and commits oneself to the practice, one will definitely not go astray. The practitioner can regulate and unblock the spider web of major and minor meridians, putting them in order. This is all clearly indicated in the book. Also included in the book are instructions on how to meditate, how to properly return to the five stems, to restore and nourish the essence, *qi*, and spirit to gradually form the pill, and how to verify from the physical and mental changes if one is successful in the initial stages. If practitioners can supplement this book with the *Yellow Court Classic* in their practice, they are likely to achieve somatic and spiritual harmony.

The [purpose of the] *Cantong Qi*'s constant explanation of the science of divinatory lines and trigrams is to provide a convenient entry point for practitioners. Ultimately, the book endeavors to lead one to the understanding that the true Dao can only be attained from realization borne out of emptiness; the rest leading up to this is nothing more than a stop-gap method. It must be said, though, that merely establishing the foundation in itself has incredible benefits. By dedicating oneself to following this trajectory one's whole life, one will eventually achieve the highest level of Daoist practice and enter into the state of unboundedness. At this point, I cannot possibly express in full, here, the meaning of the whole book, but the spirit of the *Cantong Qi* has as its objective to prevent practitioners of later generations from entering into risky circumstances through misunderstanding and blind practice. Therefore, this book was written, in the hopes that students with a karmic connection can enter the state of a Daoist immortal whose root is shared with that of Heaven and Earth.

What is regrettable is that those seeking the Dao are many, while those practicing the Dao are few. The few people who have acquired the proper oral tips have ended up living their lives in vain, all due to various life circumstances and the lack of inner cultivation. This is a real pity. Furthermore, following the Ming and Qing Dynasties, various Daoist external alchemy methods became vogue, ranging from supplementary double practice to burning lead in the cauldron. Some emphasized guarding the acupoints, while others obsessed about astral deity talismans and fasting, depriving themselves of food and sleep. If one is able to fully understand Wei Boyang's *Cantong Qi*, while referencing the annotations by the Daoist priest Zhu Yunyang, one will be able to understand the proper way of Daoist practice, without getting caught up in elaborate performances or self-deception. Therefore, it's not hard to see why the *Cantong Qi*, written with profound truth, has its place in this world. The purpose is to help people return to their original, free, and pure mind, de-rooting every dust-like bit of affliction from their mind, allowing every meditating practitioner to obtain the unified truth of heaven and humanity, handling affairs with an open mind and humility without over-doing it. Being genuine in every action is to always be in a state of peace and non-action, observing ultimate emptiness and quietude, with a sense of humanity and justice, not desiring or seeking, holding fast to moderation to achieve the Way/Dao. This is the practice method of the Qingjing Sect, one of the most important in Daoism.

CHAPTER 50

ALL TEACHINGS ARE EMPTY, ONE'S NATURE IS ALREADY COMPLETE

In my youth when I studied Daoist meditation and oral tips, I would hear from various elders the name of another Daoist patriarch, Huang Chang (Huang Yuanji). His life was colorful and miraculous, and up to this day its particulars are up for debate. According to the annals of Daoism, Huang Chang had made a name for himself during the Tang and Song Dynasties. Emperor Huizong of the Song Dynasty even ordered him to edit and compile the texts of the Daoist canon. Later, in the Yuan Dynasty he popped up again, and we then had to wait until the Qing Dynasty for him to show his face once more to the world. It's said that he continually reappeared on account of the karmic predestination he held with his disciples, to ensure the transmission of his Daoist lineage of the "Joyful Learning Parlor" to the present day. The truly fantastic stories of Huang Yuanji levitating have been passed on by generations of masters by word of mouth, and bear the seal of authenticity. It was said that finally, in the Qing Dynasty, as he stood in front of an Eight Immortals table, he levitated and disappeared from amidst his disciples. He didn't really do this to make a strong statement. He just wanted later generations to understand the heights the immortals can reach: how they can materialize and dissolve at will. However, later and modern scholars seem to have reservations about such a claim, owing to their research and academic probing and deduction into the record of Huang's discourses written during the Qing Dynasty. They simply believe that as he left the lecture hall where he had taught for 11 years, he left the last answers to his students in unmistakably plain language. Huang Yuanji would repeatedly exhort his disciples to be unwaveringly diligent in pursuing the Dao, uphold their practice, and seek confirmation of their progress. On his final day of teaching, many of his students were distraught at the idea of saying farewell, yet right before the many eyes staring at him and without uttering a further word, he vanished into thin air. As to whether the Huang Yuanji of the Yuan Dynasty and the Huang Yuanji of the Qing Dynasty were the same person, many theories have been expounded over the years. This is a point worthy of further exploration by future generations of Daoist scholars.

I want to emphasize that it isn't Huang Yuanji's levitation, but rather his practice and his essays on ethics that are really worthy of study and emulation by later generations. His *Explanation of the Dao De Jing, Recorded Sayings of the Joyful Learning Parlor*, and *Fundamental Daoist Teachings* are particularly noteworthy. It is said that the *Recorded Sayings of the Joyful Learning Parlor* are a collection of elementary teachings Huang Yuanji gave to beginner disciples and were thus not meant for publication. Later, because he had seen too many bookshops full of inauthentic books and the world was unstable, he couldn't bear to see the Great Dao kept from the world. He wished to awaken society's sense of virtue and morals. Accordingly, the book became accessible for the happiness and good fortune of common people and Daoist practitioners alike. The book's content seamlessly assimilates the three doctrines of Daoism, Confucianism, and Buddhism. The author holds none of his knowledge back and spares no effort to uplift his audience. At a glance, it seems to be a book about managing one's affairs, but upon closer reading one will gasp in astonishment at the inexhaustible gnosis found within. In the *Recorded Sayings of the Joyful Learning Parlor*, Huang Yuanji reveals that which his predecessors had not, and unleashes the torrent of his realizations upon his disciples. As the saying goes, "the authentic tradition can be held on half a piece of paper, while false teachings are the burden of a whole cart." Indeed, from ancient times until now, walking the path to immortality does not mean one must abandon one's wife and children or completely abandon one's wealth. It doesn't mean one has to travel 1,000 miles in search of a master and study with them for many years, serving under them and toiling endlessly one's entire life with, in the end, very little to show for it. In view of the many books written in a manner to send the reader tumbling into mist and fog, with obscure and abstruse doctrines for company, Mr. Yuanji wrote in a concise, comprehensive, simple, and clear style. Additionally, the practice is described in a way to suit all levels, and it can be used as a guide for both the cultivation of body and mind. The sequence of the author's exposition is a testimonial to the profundity of his cultivation:

> Unable to recite *dhāraṇī*s [a kind of Buddhist prayer/mantra] the mind must abide within the chest cavity. Since ancient times, all the oral tips of masters of the three great schools have never departed from that phrase. A cultivator of the Dao must at all times and in all places abide in purity and non-action. One does not need to contemplate emptiness for what must cease to cease. The Dao has always been natural, bereft of stillness or motion, beginning or end. If one desires for things not to be in one's mind, one must first not have one's mind in things. Don't ponder over good and evil, for what kind of person desires to know Heaven's law? Just as there is nothing more to a mirror than the light it reflects, so we should deal with things, responding only as they arise. One's wondrous awareness is originally perfect and luminous, so what is there to correct or subdue? If our eyes could see all that is illuminated, how would we keep up with details and things as miniscule as mustard seeds? The world originates in vast space, so what is there to hate or rejoice at? Although clouds move through the sky, to catch their head or tail is a futile endeavor. To force oneself to return to the natural way of things is to enter the wondrous realms of non-action.

It is unknown whether the preface was written by Huang Chang, but the whole essay reads in a very carefree way and makes for a most pleasant read. This is especially the case in the line "One's wondrous awareness is originally perfect and luminous, so what is there to correct or subdue?" If all people are originally endowed with luminous true mind, what need is there to engage in spiritual practice? The Dao is to be found within, so what need is there to seek without? Practicing meditation in search for the Dao is just like reciting a mantra or the Buddha's name; it is just a convenient means of countering delusion with an illusion. Do not be attached. Live out your days idly and your precious human life is spent in vain. I remember when my master transmitted the oral tips of Zhang Sanfeng to me and the joy it brought me. This was because from the very start the emphasis is on being natural and non-attached, until you reach a state devoid of thought. Although in some stages you direct the *qi* with your intention past the three gates, and even practice methods whereby you exit your body in spirit, in the end you must always return to emptiness till you reach the utmost of emptiness which contains the Great Dao. What is astonishing with this approach is the constant emptying out of any and all "things," and that everything Zhang Sanfeng spoke about was geared toward returning to the self-nature we all possess. Only this is the genuine goal of meditation, from the outset. After I understood this secret through my own practice, I entered a whole new perspective in the way I thought about my meditation practice. In my early years, having had indescribable admiration for Wang Yangming's spiritual resolve and Zhu Xi's teachings, I was largely influenced by their interpretations of the meaning of *ge wu zhi zhi* (格物致知), "investigating the nature of things." However, the latter's approach seemed slightly too contrived and, indeed, he ultimately made himself sick. His words "there is no reason outside the mind, and there is no object outside the mind," although simple, were very logical. The influence Wang Yangming received from Lu Jiuyuan was actually very deep. Ultimately, he deeply felt that the views of Cheng Yi and Zhu Xi were too complicated and abstruse. He asserted the reasoning that the mind is all things;

furthermore, it must embrace all things Nature produces. Taking it another step forward, the cultivator must in body and spirit abide by the principle of unity of understanding and enactment, and of the unity of man and Heaven.

This was when I was about 20 years old, but as I got older I delved into even more books on the nature of the mind, the main points, and Daoist and Buddhist tomes. I am quite convinced that even though the study of the School of Principles can lead to the understanding Wang Yangming spoke of, it is not the ultimate state. Latecomers such as modern Confucianists Xiong Shili and Mou Zongsan were also influenced by his thought, and even filially upheld and passed down his system, of which I am deeply admiring. Yet, why did the Buddha, after reaching enlightenment, gazing into the stars, fearlessly proclaiming and flourishing his doctrine for 49 years, then say in the end that he had not once spoken a word? The crux is expressed in few words. Daoism has existed for about 5,000 years and has seen over 100 schools sprout within it, and yet they too always return to one's self-nature. Therefore, in this short life, the thing we must urgently seek to find must be this thing we all possess to begin with, this thing that need not be sought without and that is complete in itself. What other pith instruction is needed? This pith instruction is neither within, nor without; all we must strive to comprehend is that all forms and phenomena are all void of true reality, so how are we to ever grasp or obtain them? In the end, all I can offer are these few words to fellow practitioners with a karmic connection. If you were to ask me about the fruit of half a life of meditation, I would only ashamedly share these verses of the sixth patriarch Huineng to create an auspicious karmic connection: "What a wonder! This self-nature is originally pure in itself, neither born nor extinguishing! What a wonder! This self-nature is originally complete in itself, unmoving! What a wonder! This self-nature can give rise to all myriad phenomena!"

Master Huineng had an enlightenment experience upon reading the *Diamond Sutra*. The main points of the *Diamond Sutra* are numerous: if one wanted to apply them in one's meditation and reach the highest level, one must first reach the state of "non-abiding," sitting without sitting. However, one must take note that non-abiding is not the ultimate state of emptiness. It's not that one cannot "sit" per se; it's just that one must not be particularly attached to the act of "sitting" in itself. As soon as the thought of wanting to sit arises in one's mind, then one is attached to an "abode," and once we abide in something, we fall into the realm of form and the aggregates. You could sit immovable in this way for 1,000 years, or even 10,000 like the trees and stones, but your practice would prove fruitless.

Genuine meditation is to sit until you let go completely of both body and mind, and then there will be no concern about having numb legs or moving around. You will be like water. All waters find the ocean, without provenance or destination: this is the state of the *Tathāgatas.*[1] Were there to be a conclusive note on the topic of meditation, that would be it. Some people ask me if there is a distinction between before and after meditation. In my humble opinion, if we have meditated for a certain time and still cling to the before and after of our sessions, we are in fact clinging to existence and non-existence. To uphold the *Diamond Sutra*'s exhortation to "guard well our thoughts," there can be no differentiation between "before" and "after," nor any guarding of acupoints or application of pith instructions, nor in fact the self-righteous belief that one will one day transcend one's physical state and reach the truth. To guard our thoughts well until all abides without abiding, is calm without calm, is letting go without letting go of—this is truly the unsurpassed, marvelous method of melding all activities, still or in motion, into one's meditation practice. If you can reach this state, you have transcended that of the immortals; your mind and actions reside in emptiness, and you attain the purity of your self-nature, giving rise to the equanimity of a Buddha, to the

---

1   *Tathāgata* (singular): A Pali word, literally meaning "Thus Come One," but also "one who is beyond all coming and going, all phenomena." A common epithet for Shakyamuni Buddha, and for all Buddhas in general.

equality of *samsāra* and Nirvana. These are the humble views I have developed through a lifelong journey of meditation started in my youth, through the traditions of Daoism, Buddhism, Chan, and Vajrayana, and is also the direction I wish to direct the future of my endeavors. I humbly implore those of greater capacity to please amend my writing.

Note: *The stories in this book are based on real people and real events. Some people's names have been changed to aliases. Any reference to current people/events is purely coincidental.*

PART 2

PRACTICE GUIDE AND EXERCISES

As with any type of physical activity, if you suffer from high blood pressure or heart disease, have had major surgery, or have any kind of mental illness or other chronic conditions, we recommend you check with your physician before practicing the following exercises.

The "12-Step Brocade"— *Qi* Bathing Techniques for Longevity

Benefits

This practice method arose from the Daoist School of Complete Reality. It is of particular benefit for the elderly and for those recovering after an illness. It can also be used after meditation to help ensure that the meridians are kept open and the *qi* can circulate unobstructed. This is a very effective set of Daoist exercises: just by practicing these alone, one can experience the benefit of having *qi* flow freely throughout the whole body, akin to an effective meditation session. Paired with the "Exhaling the Old and Inhaling the New"[1] practice and breath regulation, and combined with movements of the muscles, tendons, and bones, it ensures there will be no stagnant *qi* along the practitioner's eight extraordinary meridians. Beginners on the path of meditation can practice this set before or after meditating. The balanced combination of movement and stillness will be of natural benefit to one's overall health, well-being, and *qi* cultivation, regulating the spirit, replenishing the essence, and transforming *qi*.

Appropriate location for practice

Ideally, find a place with good airflow and away from too much noise, in order to practice more effectively.

---

1   A conscious way of breathing that helps purge the body from impurities. One imagines dirty *qi* being expelled during exhalation, and pure, nourishing *qi* being absorbed during inhalation.

While practicing this set of exercises, as you inhale, curl the tongue upward and rest it on the area where the top teeth and palate meet. Very lightly clench the perineum, and very gently grip the floor with the soles of your feet. Your entire body and mind, however, must remain completely relaxed, devoid of any psychophysical strain or tension. As you exhale, curl the tongue downward, resting it just behind the bottom teeth, relaxing the soles of the feet and perineum at the same time.

Preparatory Stance

1. Stand with feet shoulder-width apart. Regulate the breath 7 times until the body is completely relaxed (Figure 1).

2. Imagine two streams of *qi* at the *yongquan* points on the soles of the feet. Gently activate your intention and let your knees bend, crouching slightly. The knees must not reach further than the tips of the toes.

3. Both arms lift naturally and gently to the same height as the *tanzhong* acupoint in the center of the chest, curving as if holding a large tree trunk. Adjust the breath until comfortable (Figure 2).

4. Breathe in and out a total of 21 times, curling the tongue upward toward the palate just behind the top teeth while inhaling, curling it down to rest behind the bottom teeth when exhaling. There is no need to pay attention to the soles of the feet or the perineum at this time.

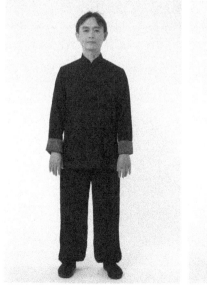
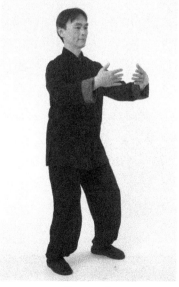

FIGURE 1   FIGURE 2

1ST EXERCISE

1. Stand with feet shoulder-width apart, and let the arms hang beside the thighs (Figure 1.1).

2. Lift the arms out to the left and right, palms facing forward, to the height of the shoulders. As the arms rise, slowly and gently inhale (Figure 1.2).

3. From here, move the arms inward and cross them in front of the chest, left arm on top, right hand below. Both hands pat the shoulders as if in a self-embrace (Figure 1.3). Then relax and return the arms out to the sides.

4. Again, cross the arms in front of the chest, this time with the right arm above and the left below, and with the hands again patting each shoulder (Figure 1.4). Then relax and return the arms out to the sides.

5. Repeat both actions 7 times each. Keep the breathing relaxed and unforced while doing this exercise. There is no need to pay attention to the tongue, feet or perineum—just keep everything natural.

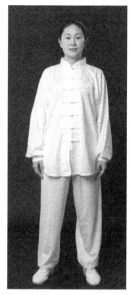
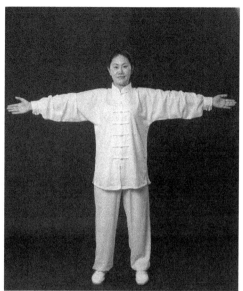

FIGURE 1.1   FIGURE 1.2

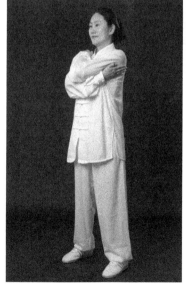
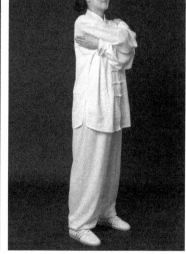

FIGURE 1.3   FIGURE 1.4

2ND EXERCISE

1. Maintain the same posture as in the previous exercise, arms swinging back and forth, crossing and embracing and patting the sides of the shoulders; only this time, as the arms cross, the knees should bend slightly, as in the preparatory posting exercise, making sure the knees do not reach beyond the toes. Inhale as you crouch, exhale as you straighten the knees.

2. Repeat the cycle 7 times (Figures 2.1 to 2.3).

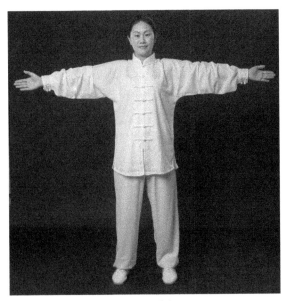

FIGURE 2.1

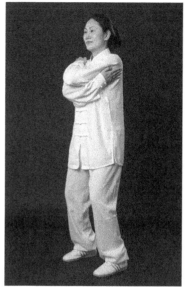

FIGURE 2.2

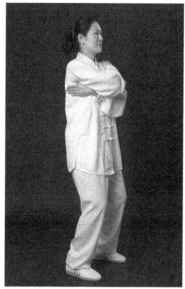

FIGURE 2.3

3rd Exercise

1. Stand with feet shoulder-width apart. Twist the upper body back and forth, letting the arms swing as if they were a hand drum, patting the opposite shoulder and hip at each turn.

2. As the upper body twists to the left, the right palm pats the left shoulder while the back of the left hand pats the right hip, and vice versa. Repeat the action 7 times on each side (Figures 3.1 to 3.5). Breathe naturally as you practice this form. There's no need to pay attention to the tongue, feet, or perineum—just keep everything relaxed and natural.

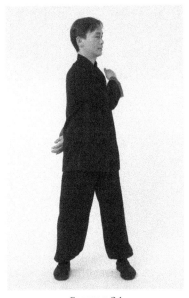 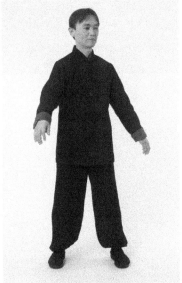

FIGURE 3.1   FIGURE 3.2

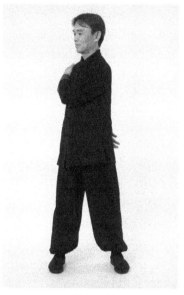

FIGURE 3.3

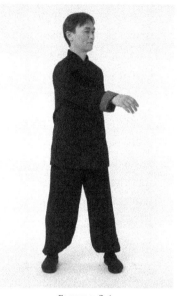

FIGURE 3.4

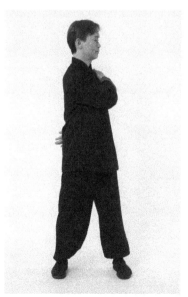

FIGURE 3.5

4TH EXERCISE

1. Stand and relax, with feet shoulder-width apart. Overlap the hands over the lower abdomen, thumbs crossing, and imagine a *taiji* symbol sitting on the *dantian*. As the hands slightly press the abdomen, draw full circles on top of the *dantian*, first in a clockwise direction, 36 times, then counterclockwise, 36 times (Figure 4.1).

2. After this, inhale and curl the tongue up behind the top teeth, while pressing the toes into the ground and lifting the heels, and moving the hands upward, palms up (Figure 4.2). As the hands pass the *tanzhong* area, turn them so the palms continue to face up (Figures 4.3 and 4.4). Then stretch the arms upward, vertically, as if pushing the sky (Figure 4.5).

3. Exhale as the hands move apart and downward, like a bird slowly bringing its wings back to the body. Gradually bring the arms back to the sides of the legs, as the heels slowly and gently reach back down to the ground (Figure 4.6).

4. Repeat the actions in Steps 2 and 3 a total of 7 times.

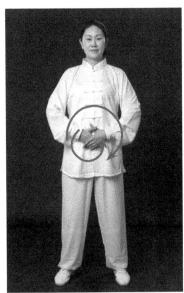

FIGURE 4.1

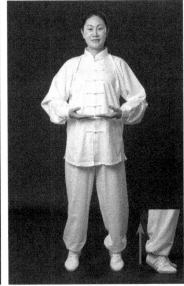

FIGURE 4.2

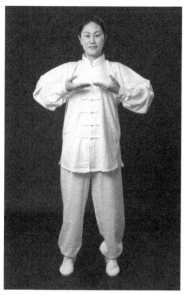

FIGURE 4.3

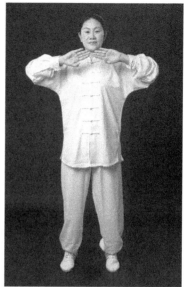

FIGURE 4.4

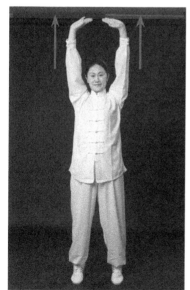

FIGURE 4.5

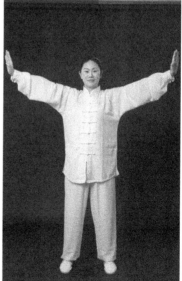

FIGURE 4.6

5TH EXERCISE

1. Stand with feet shoulder-width apart. Clap the hands together 3 times (Figures 5.1 and 5.2), then rub them until hot (Figure 5.3).

2. Place the palms flat on the forehead and rub it, then move on to the cheeks and then the back of the head (Figures 5.4 and 5.5).

3. Clap the hands again and rub them until hot, then use the heat to rub the chest area, kidneys and lower back, buttocks, down the medial side of the thighs, then the back of the thighs and lower legs, all the way until comfortable (Figures 5.6 to 5.11).

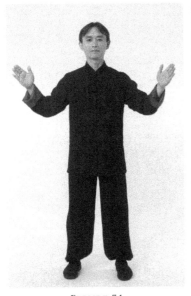
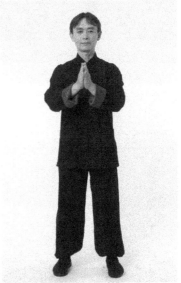

FIGURE 5.1   FIGURE 5.2

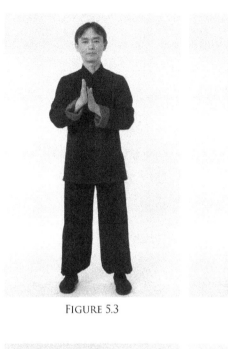

FIGURE 5.3

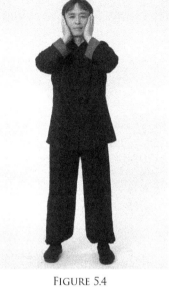

FIGURE 5.4

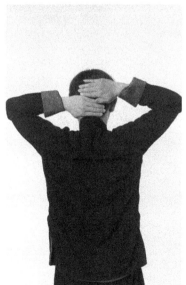

FIGURE 5.5

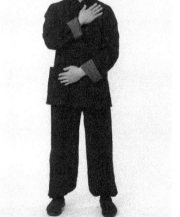

FIGURE 5.6

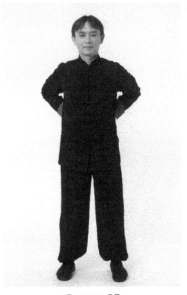

FIGURE 5.7

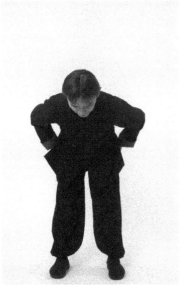

FIGURE 5.8

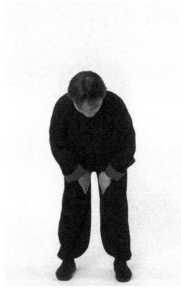

FIGURE 5.9

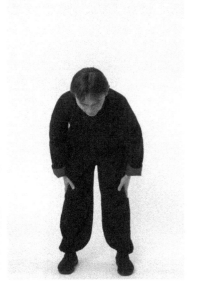

FIGURE 5.10

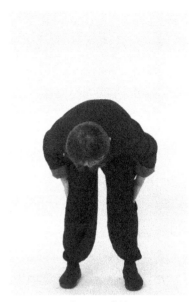

FIGURE 5.11

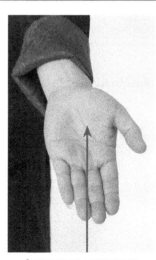

When rubbing the hands, imagine the *laogong* acupoint in the palm of the hands emitting a scorching heat like that of a bright sun.

LAOGONG ACUPOINT

6TH EXERCISE

1. Stand with feet shoulder-width apart. Breathe naturally (Figure 6.1).

2. Lean the upper body slightly backward. As you lean, open the arms to the sides and back, as if drawing a large circle in the air. As the upper body returns to vertical, the arms follow, then continue forward, bringing the upper body slowly into a forward bend (Figures 6.2 to 6.5).

3. Breathe in as you lean back, and breathe out as you come back to the vertical axis and bend forward. Repeat the cycle 7 times.

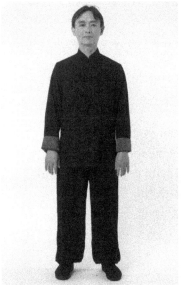

FIGURE 6.1

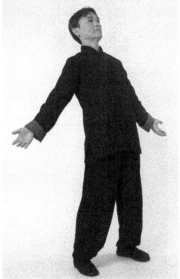

FIGURE 6.2

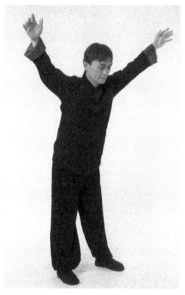

FIGURE 6.3

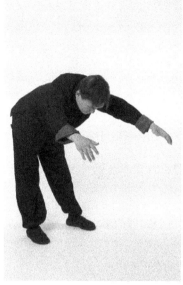

FIGURE 6.4

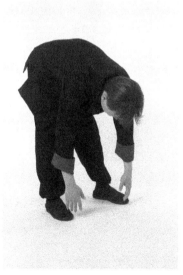

FIGURE 6.5

7th Exercise

1. Stand with feet shoulder-width apart. Bring the hands together, one on top of the other, thumbs lightly touching, in front of the *dantian*. Relax and regulate the breath 3 to 7 times (Figure 7.1).

2. As you slowly inhale, gently lift the hands up to the *tanzhong* acupoint in the middle of the sternum, then inhale completely as you expand the chest, palms now facing forward (Figures 7.2 and 7.3).

3. Push and extend the arms and hands forward, then out to the sides, parallel to the ground, as if gliding on water (Figures 7.4 and 7.5). Exhale naturally, then bend the upper body forward, as if to pick something up, making sure the knees do not bend. The hands touch the floor while the arms are extended vertically.

4. Maintain the forward bend and breathe naturally as the left and right arm begin to move up and down, vertically, in alternating fashion, a number of times (Figure 7.6). After this, begin swinging the arms to touch the left leg, then the right leg (Figure 7.7). Your intention is not to use force; rather be completely relaxed, swinging like a rope moving to and fro in the blowing wind. Repeat the cycle of three motions (vertical arms up and down touching the ground, swinging left, swinging right) 3 to 7 times.

5. Return the upper body to the original standing position, with the arms and hands the same, palms one on top of the other facing upward (Figure 7.1). Regulate the breath, in 3 to 7 breath cycles.

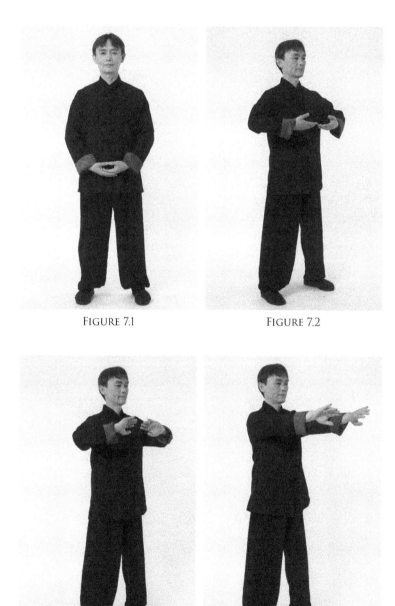

FIGURE 7.1

FIGURE 7.2

FIGURE 7.3

FIGURE 7.4

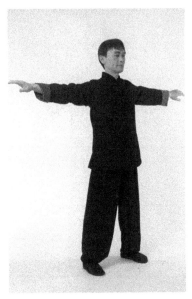

FIGURE 7.5

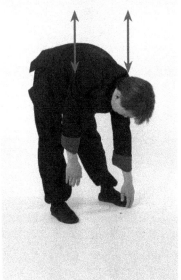

FIGURE 7.6

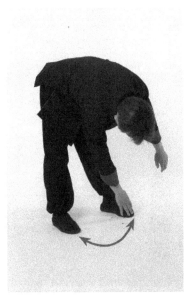

FIGURE 7.7

8TH EXERCISE

1. Stand with feet shoulder-width apart. Regulate the breath until comfortable and natural (Figure 8.1).

2. Place both hands on your hips, and prepare to do a twisting motion with the neck. First, tilt your head up and back, looking up, then bow it forward, looking down. Repeat this 7 times (Figure 8.2). Then tilt the head left and right, ear toward the shoulder, and repeat 7 times (Figure 8.3). Finally, rotate the head clockwise 360°, then counterclockwise, and repeat 7 times both ways (Figure 8.4).

3. Lift both arms out to the sides, palms facing downward, and rotate the trunk (Figure 8.5). First turn the whole upper body to the left until you can't turn any further (Figure 8.6). Return to the neutral forward-facing stance. Inhale as you turn to the left, exhale as you return to the front.

4. Inhale again as you turn to the right in the same manner (Figure 8.6). Exhale as you return facing forward. Repeat the cycle left and right a total of 7 times.

5. Slowly inhale as you squat down, as if sitting on a low bench, keeping the upper body vertical, until your glutes and knees are level (Figure 8.7). Exhale, then smoothly push the upper body back up to standing. Repeat this movement 7 times.

Reminder: When turning the upper body, the lower body from the waist downward remains motionless.

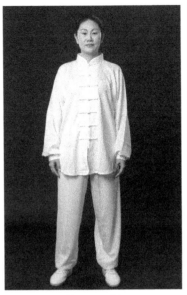

FIGURE 8.1

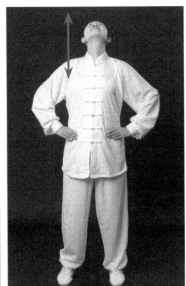

FIGURE 8.2

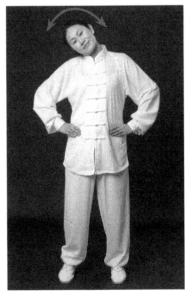

FIGURE 8.3

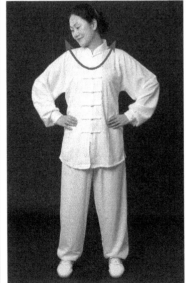

FIGURE 8.4

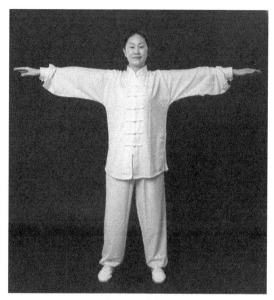

FIGURE 8.5

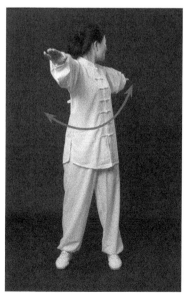

FIGURE 8.6

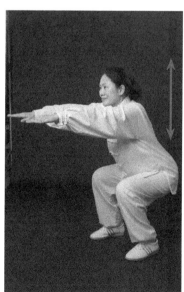

FIGURE 8.7

9TH EXERCISE

1. Stand with feet shoulder-width apart. Regulate the breath until smooth and comfortable.

2. Clap the hands 3 times (Figure 9.1). Rub the palms together until hot (Figure 9.2). Place the palms on the lower back and rub the kidney area in a circular fashion, 36 times (Figure 9.3).

3. Clap the hands again, rub the palms until hot, then massage the glutes, the inner and outer thighs, and continue down to the calves and lower legs (Figures 9.4 to 9.7).

4. Sit on the ground, clap the hands again and rub them until hot (Figure 9.8). Massage the *yongquan* points on the soles of both feet (Figure 9.9).

5. Use your thumbs to massage the acupoints between your metatarsals, using a comfortable amount of pressure, pressing outward toward the toes (Figure 9.10).

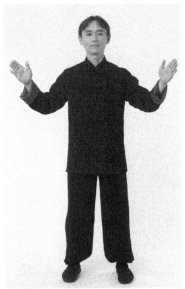

FIGURE 9.1

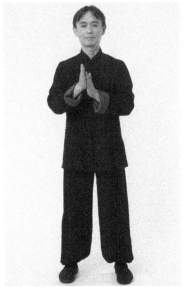

FIGURE 9.2

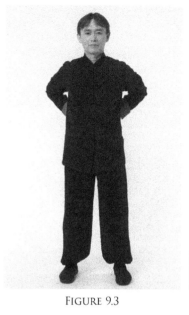

FIGURE 9.3

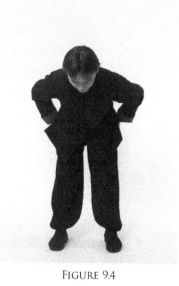

FIGURE 9.4

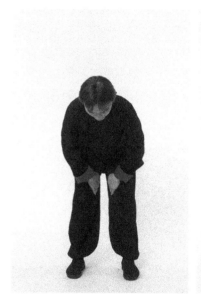

FIGURE 9.5

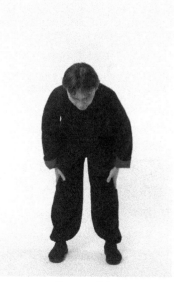

FIGURE 9.6

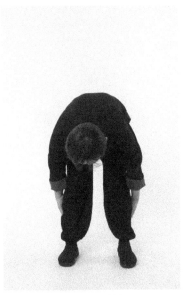

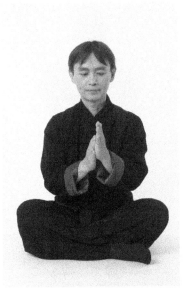

FIGURE 9.7

FIGURE 9.8

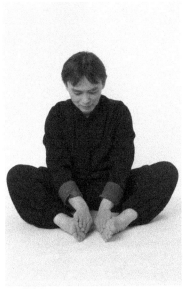

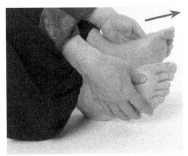

FIGURE 9.9

FIGURE 9.10

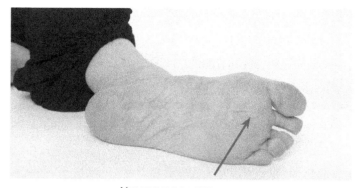

YONGQUAN ACUPOINT

10TH EXERCISE

1. Stand with feet shoulder-width apart. Regulate the breath until naturally comfortable (Figure 10.1).

2. Visualize the space in front of you as a void of perfect blue color, like a sunny, cloudless sky. An abundance of all five elements of the universe fill the void, transforming into the five colors (red, yellow, white, green, blue), which create a rainbow-like atmosphere.

3. Inhale, as you imagine all the *qi* of Heaven and Earth and the five auspicious colors combining together, then being absorbed from the crown of the head, to fill your whole body completely.

4. As you bend the upper body forward about 90°, exhale with force and make the sound "HA!", imagining that all the turbid, uncomfortable *qi* inside the body is expelled with the exhalation, coming out as gray smoke (Figure 10.2).

5. Having exhaled completely, return the body to the original standing position as you inhale, then repeat the whole cycle 7 times.

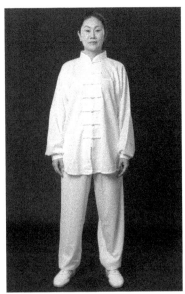 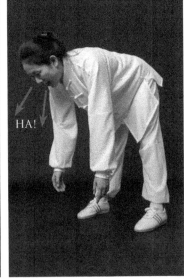

FIGURE 10.1   FIGURE 10.2

11TH EXERCISE

1. Stand with feet shoulder-width apart. Regulate the breath until smooth and comfortable (Figure 11.1).

2. Inhale, and raise the hands up in front of the body, palms up (Figures 11.2 to 11.4). Do this while raising the heels off the floor (Figure 11.5). As the hands reach the head, turn them, extending the arms vertically with palms facing the sky, as if lifting the Heavens.

3. Face upward, open your eyes as wide as possible and look into the sky above you, while exhaling with force and making the sound "HA!", imagining that all the turbid *qi* inside the body is thus expelled (Figure 11.6).

4. Extend the arms out to the side and downward, while returning the heels back down to the floor (Figure 11.7).

5. Repeat the cycle 7 times.

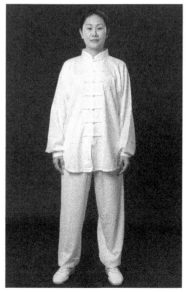

FIGURE 11.1

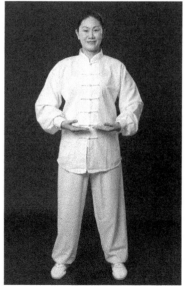

FIGURE 11.2

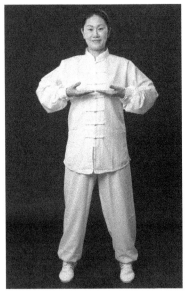

FIGURE 11.3

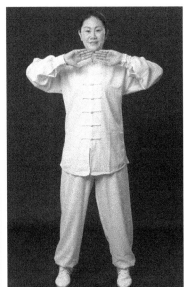

FIGURE 11.4

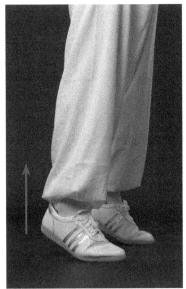

FIGURE 11.5

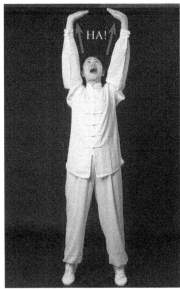

FIGURE 11.6

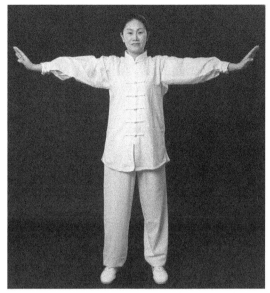

FIGURE 11.7

12th Exercise

1. Stand with feet shoulder-width apart. Breathe naturally, completely relaxing the mind and body (Figure 12.1).

2. Close your eyes. Move the eyeballs behind the lids left to right 7 to 21 times; then up and down 7 to 21 times; then rotate them 360° (Figure 12.2).

3. Rub your palms together, place them evenly on your face to apply warmth, then massage downward from the forehead to the chin until comfortable, a minimum of 7 times (Figure 12.3).

4. Clack your teeth together, making a clacking sound as the upper and lower teeth hit each other. Do this 7 to 36 times.

5. Clap your hands 3 times, rub them together, then use the hands to massage the back of the head, the nape, the chest and back, all the way down to the lower legs. Massage at will, until comfortable (Figures 12.4 to 12.8).

6. Return to the original standing position, feet shoulder-width apart. Allow the breath to return to its natural, comfortable rhythm (Figure 12.1).

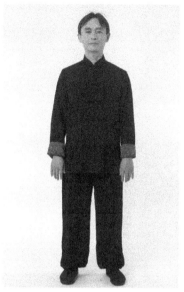

FIGURE 12.1

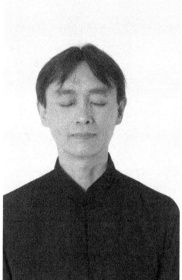

FIGURE 12.2

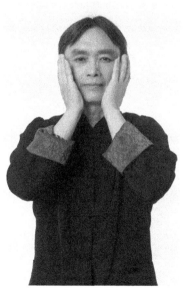

FIGURE 12.3

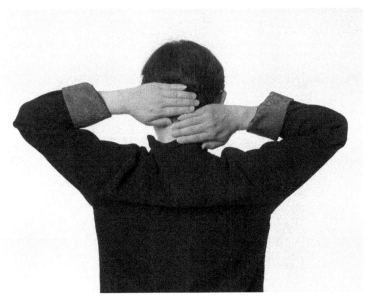

FIGURE 12.4

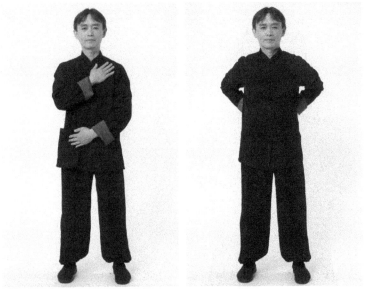

FIGURE 12.5   FIGURE 12.6

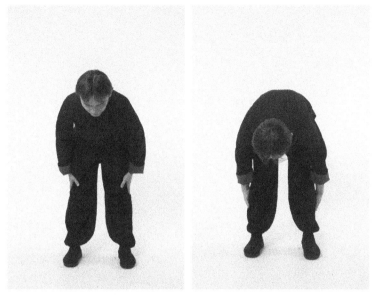

FIGURE 12.7   FIGURE 12.8

"Eight Pieces of Brocade"

Benefits

These eight movements make up one set of exercises for the body. The entire set is simple, easy to remember, and the exercise intensity is moderate. Through movement of the body, control of the breath, and in coordination with your intention, you can nourish the *yin* and benefit the *yang* energies of your body, strengthen your foundation, free up the channels and meridians of the body, enhance circulation of the blood and other bodily fluids, and calm the mind, among other benefits, all leading to enhanced functioning of all internal organs and systems.

Note: When doing seated practice, the relaxation method is nearly identical to that used when doing the standing relaxation method; however, it is best to sit in "double lotus."

1. Before beginning to practice, relax until the *laogong* points in the center of the palms feel slightly warm and swollen.

2. Pairing this set of exercises with seated meditation will enhance their effect. Do not practice this exercise when you feel hungry, or when feeling very full after a large meal.

3. Before beginning, you can first drink a glass of warm water, allowing the body to eliminate internal waste more efficiently after the practice.

4. Perform each exercise as slowly and comfortably as possible.

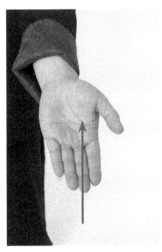

LAOGONG ACUPOINT

Preliminary Exercise

1. Stand with feet shoulder-width apart. Relax the body completely, from the *niwangong* acupoint on the top of the head down to the *yongquan* point on the bottom of the feet. Relax every cell, follicle, internal organ, channel, acupoint, all your skin and bones, etc. Feel relaxation completely permeating every corner, nook, and cranny you can think of in your body. Adjust the breath until it is comfortable.

2. When inhaling, curl the tongue up to the back of the palate; when exhaling, curl it down to touch the floor of the mouth.

3. Keep a joyful mind and body, and a smile on your face.

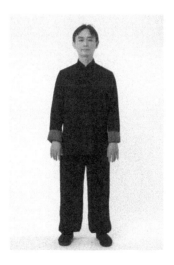

1ST EXERCISE: "TWO HANDS HOLDING UP THE SKY, ALIGNING THE TRIPLE BURNER"

1. Stand with feet shoulder-width apart. Regulate the breath until comfortable (Figure 1.1).

2. Inhale and bring the hands forward with fingers interlocked (Figure 1.2). With the palms facing up, slowly raise the hands. As they pass the lower jaw, turn them so the palms continue facing upward (Figures 1.3 and 1.4). Then straighten the arms toward the sky, stretching them behind the ears (Figure 1.5).

3. Exhale, release the hands and slowly lower the arms to the sides, palms facing downward (Figures 1.6 and 1.7).

4. Repeat Steps 2 to 3 a total of 7 times, then return to the starting position (Figure 1.1).

Reminder: Stretch the arms overhead behind the ears, allowing the meridians to open. Inhale as the hands rise, exhale through the mouth as they lower.

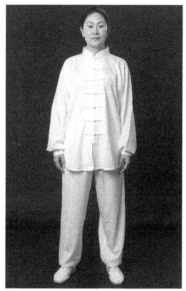

FIGURE 1.1

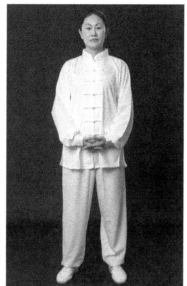

FIGURE 1.2

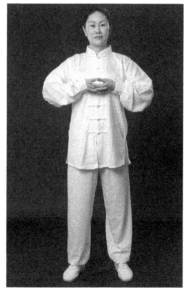

FIGURE 1.3

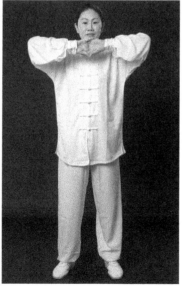

FIGURE 1.4

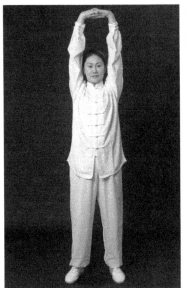

FIGURE 1.5

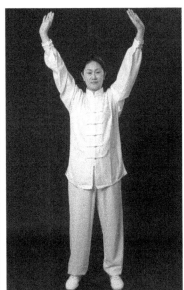

FIGURE 1.6

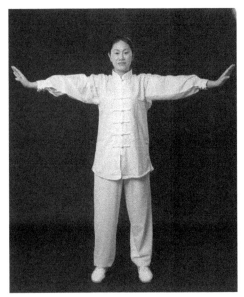

FIGURE 1.7

2nd Exercise: "Drawing the Bow Left and Right, Like a Condor"

1. Stand with feet shoulder-width apart. Regulate the breath until comfortable and even (Figure 2.1).

2. With the arms at the sides of the body, clench the hands into fists, while stepping out with one foot to widen your stance, and squat down as if assuming the horse stance posting form. The hands will now be to the sides of the waist, fists clenched (Figure 2.2).

3. Raise the arms to the chest, crossing the forearms one in front of the other (Figure 2.3).

4. Inhale and loosen the fists. As your head turns to the left, stretch the left arm out to the left side, horizontally, with the *hukou* acupoint[1] facing up. The right arm comes up to the height of the shoulder, with the hand placed below the right ear as if shooting an arrow. The eyes open wide and glare through the *hukou*, out into the distance (Figure 2.4).

5. Exhale and return the arms in front of the chest, hands clenched into fists, forearms crossing (Figure 2.5).

6. Inhale, loosen the fists, and draw the bow and arrow as in Step 4, but to the right side (Figure 2.6). Then exhale and return the arms in front of the chest, hands clenched into fists, forearms crossing (Figure 2.3).

7. Repeat Steps 4 to 6 a total of 7 times, then return to the starting position (Figure 2.1).

Reminder: The eyes should look out beyond the *hukou* acupoint, wide open, to a distant place. Inhale all the way from the arms opening in opposite directions to the eyes opening wide; exhale as the arms return to the chest.

---

1   虎口: The "tiger's mouth," an acupoint on the webbing between thumb and index fingers.

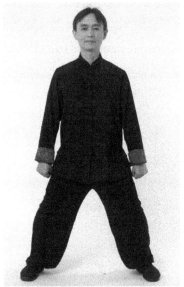

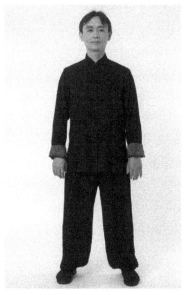

Figure 2.1

Figure 2.2

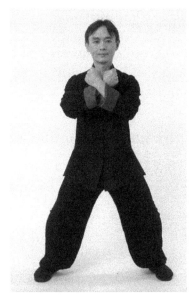

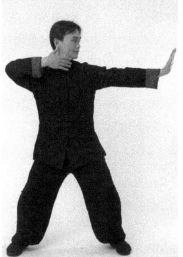

Figure 2.3

Figure 2.4

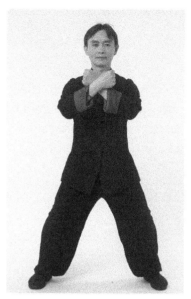

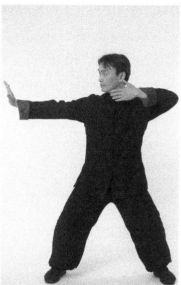

Figure 2.5

Figure 2.6

3RD EXERCISE: "SINGLE ARM STRETCHES TO REJUVENATE SPLEEN AND STOMACH"

1. Stand with feet shoulder-width apart. Regulate the breath until comfortable and even (Figure 3.1).

2. Inhale and raise the hands with palms up in front of the trunk, to the level of the *tanzhong* (Figures 3.2 and 3.3). As you exhale, the right hand turns over as the right arm stretches upward, while the left arm stretches downward, the palm facing the earth (Figures 3.4 and 3.5).

3. As you inhale, slowly return both hands toward the *tanzhong* (Figure 3.6). Then exhale and switch hands, so that as the left arm stretches upward, the right hand pushes down toward the ground (Figures 3.7 and 3.8).

4. Repeat Steps 2 and 3 a total of 7 times. Then return to the starting position (Figures 3.9, 3.10, and 3.1).

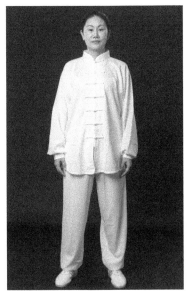 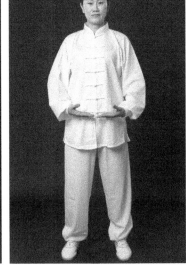

FIGURE 3.1   FIGURE 3.2

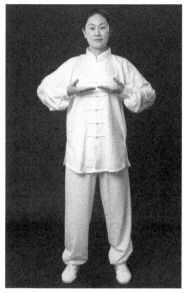

FIGURE 3.3

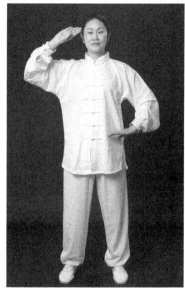

FIGURE 3.4

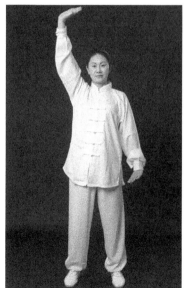

FIGURE 3.5

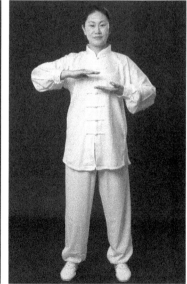

FIGURE 3.6

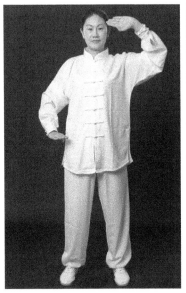

Figure 3.7

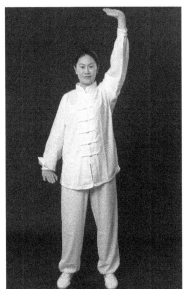

Figure 3.8

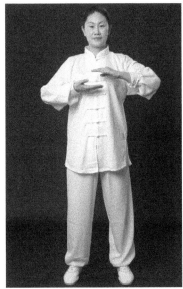

Figure 3.9

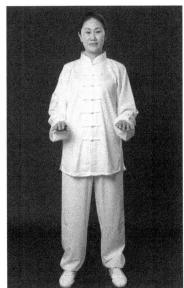

Figure 3.10

4th Exercise: "Seven Jolts to Eliminate All Illness"

1. Stand with feet shoulder-width apart. Regulate the breath until comfortable and even (Figure 4.1).

2. Draw the legs together, heels touching, toes outward, and rest the arms on your sides (Figure 4.2).

3. Inhale and lift the heels up, as the hands rise upward with palms up to the *tanzhong* (Figures 4.3 and 4.4). Then flip the palms downward and move the hands to the sides of the body (Figure 4.5).

4. As you exhale smoothly from the mouth, use force to emit the sound "HA!" as you drop the heels back to the ground, while you press the hands downward, touching the sides of the body, until they're back beside the outer thighs (Figure 4.6).

5. Repeat Steps 3 to 6 a total of 7 times, then return to the starting position.

Reminder: As hands rise to the *tanzhong*, the chest expands. As the palms press down, keep them touching the body all the way to the thighs. Use force as you exhale "HA!" to expel all turbid *qi*.

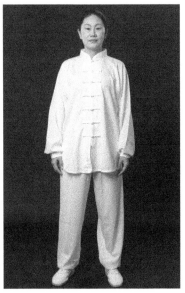

FIGURE 4.1

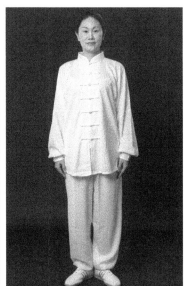

FIGURE 4.2

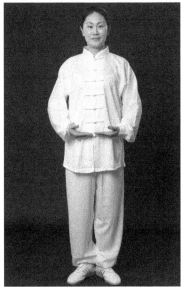

FIGURE 4.3

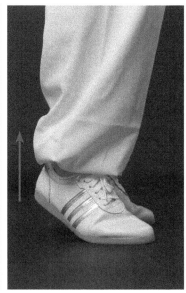

FIGURE 4.4

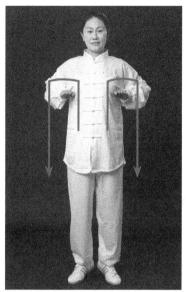

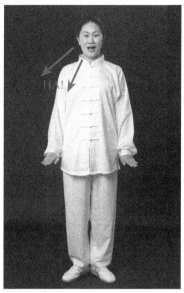

FIGURE 4.5   FIGURE 4.6

5th Exercise: "Withdraw the Fists and Glare to Increase Vigor"

1. Stand with feet shoulder-width apart. Regulate the breath until comfortable and even (Figure 5.1).

2. Step out to beyond shoulder width, clench your fists and place them by the waist, palms up, as you take a breath in (Figure 5.2).

3. Exhale as the right fist opens, and the palm pushes straight forward with force, while you crouch into horse stance (Figure 5.3).

4. Rotate your outstretched right palm to the right in a semicircle (Figures 5.4 and 5.5). Then clench the fist again, and return it to the side of the waist, palm up, as you inhale and straighten the knees. After the fist is back beside the waist, exhale (Figure 5.6).

5. Take a breath in, then exhale as you unclench the left fist, pressing the palm straight forward with force, as if pushing someone, while you squat into horse stance again (Figure 5.7).

6. Rotate the outstretched left palm to the left in a semicircle (Figures 5.8 and 5.9). Then clench the fist again, and return it to the side of the waist, palm up, as you inhale and straighten the knees. After the fist is back to the waist, exhale (Figure 5.10).

7. Repeat the sequence of movements 7 times, then return to the starting position (Figure 5.1).

Reminder: As you push the hand out, use force and glare with eyes wide open, exerting force all the way to each fingertip. The exercise must be performed to the fullest for it to be beneficial.

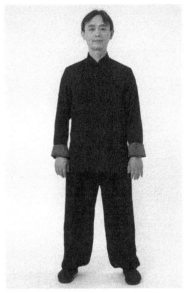

FIGURE 5.1

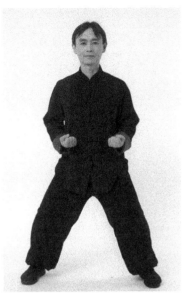

FIGURE 5.2

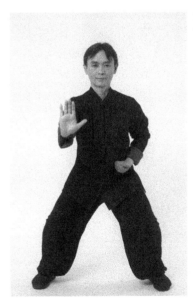

FIGURE 5.3

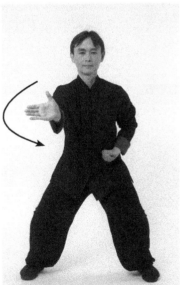

FIGURE 5.4

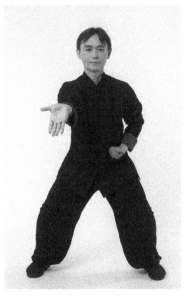

Figure 5.5

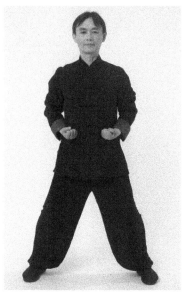

Figure 5.6

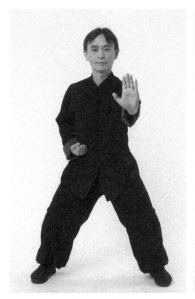

Figure 5.7

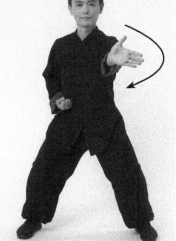

Figure 5.8

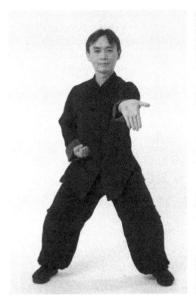 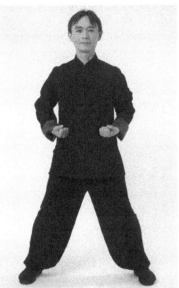

FIGURE 5.9   FIGURE 5.10

6th Exercise: "Looking Back at Your Illnesses"

1. Stand with feet shoulder-width apart. Regulate the breath until smooth and even (Figure 6.1).

2. Place your arms akimbo, hands above the hips, *hukou* and thumbs facing down (Figure 6.2).

3. Inhale and press the chin close to the body (Figure 6.3). Then slowly turn the head to the right shoulder, eyes looking back toward the right heel (Figure 6.4). Exhale, and slowly return the head to the front, as the chin keeps pressing against the body (Figure 6.5).

4. Inhale and move the head toward the left shoulder, chin pressing down, as you try to look toward the left heel (Figures 6.6 and 6.7). Then exhale, bringing the head back forward.

5. Repeat Steps 3 and 4 a total of 7 times, then return to the starting position (Figure 6.1).

> Reminder: When inhaling and exhaling, keep the chin touching the chest at all times.

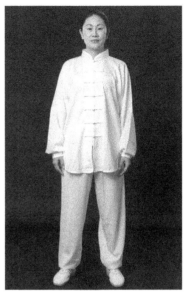

FIGURE 6.1

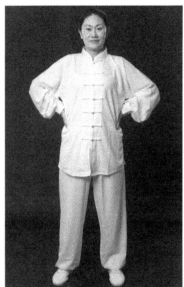

FIGURE 6.2

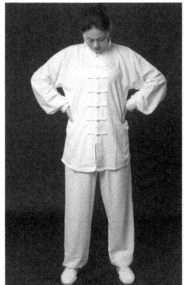

FIGURE 6.3

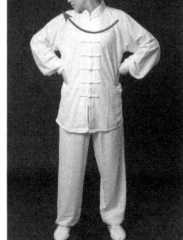

FIGURE 6.4

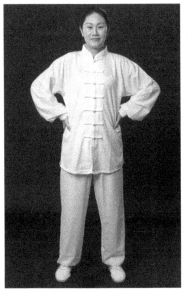

FIGURE 6.5

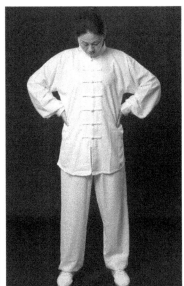

FIGURE 6.6

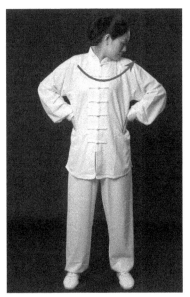

FIGURE 6.7

7th Exercise: "Shake the Head and Wag the Tail to Get Rid of Heart Fire"

1. Stand with feet shoulder-width apart. Regulate the breath until smooth and even (Figure 7.1).

2. Step out to a stance wider than your shoulders, legs crouching as in horse stance, with the palms of the hands on each knee (Figure 7.2).

3. Breathe in, then breathe out, while you slowly bring the right shoulder to the left knee (Figure 7.3). Inhale, then continue the circle, panning the upper body to the front while exhaling, then back up to complete the circle. The head is always aligned with the straight spine, moving 360° back to the horse stance in Step 2 (Figures 7.4 to 7.6).

4. Inhale again, then exhale as you slowly bring the left shoulder to the right knee (Figure 7.7). Draw a circle with the upper body as before (Figures 7.8 to 7.10). As you turn the body, make sure the hips, groin, and buttocks twist and move in unison with the upper body (Figure 7.11).

5. After drawing circles to the left and right 7 times, return to the starting position (Figure 7.1).

Reminder: Try your best to bring your shoulder all the way to your knee, while your feet stand firm and motionless. As you perform the exercise, your eyes follow the direction of the movement, looking outward.

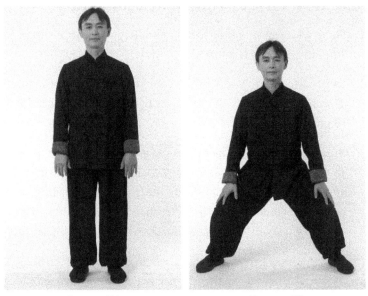

FIGURE 7.1   FIGURE 7.2

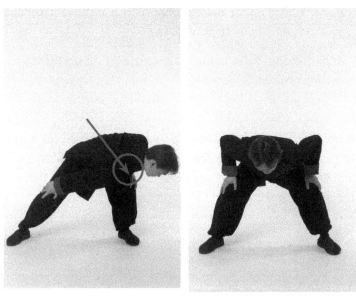

FIGURE 7.3   FIGURE 7.4

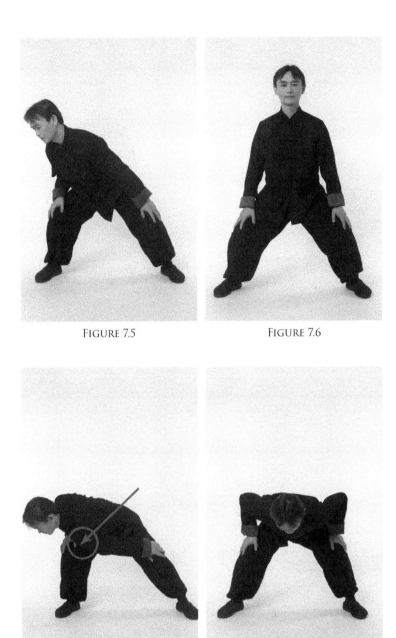

FIGURE 7.5

FIGURE 7.6

FIGURE 7.7

FIGURE 7.8

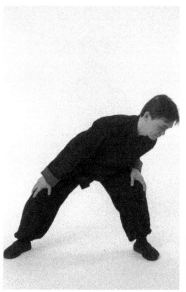

FIGURE 7.9

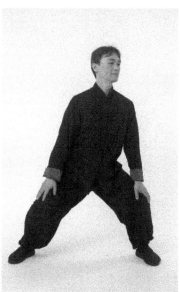

FIGURE 7.10

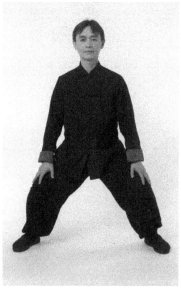

FIGURE 7.11

8th Exercise: "Grabbing the Feet with Two Hands to Strengthen the Lower Back"

1. Stand with feet shoulder-width apart. Regulate the breath until comfortable and even (Figure 8.1).

2. Place the hands one on top of the other, palms up, comfortably in front of the two legs, by the *dantian* (Figure 8.2).

3. Inhale and slowly raise the hands, palms up. As they reach the chin, turn the palms to press up as you stretch the arms upward and exhale (Figures 8.3 to 8.5).

4. Inhale, then with arms and hands straight, bow forward, bending at the waist as you exhale. Reach the hands to the tips of your toes, keeping your legs straight (Figures 8.6 to 8.8).

5. Inhale as you return to standing, bring the two hands to overlap in front of the *dantian*, then exhale (Figure 8.2).

6. Repeat Steps 3 to 5 a total of 7 times, then return to the initial standing posture (Figure 8.1).

Reminder: As the arms move downward, exhale completely, until empty. Once all the air is out, pause for half a second to a second, then inhale back up.

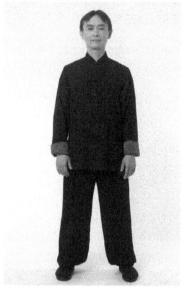

FIGURE 8.1

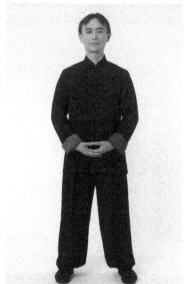

FIGURE 8.2

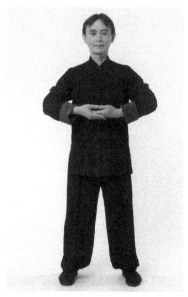

FIGURE 8.3

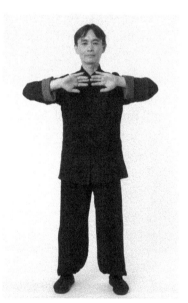

FIGURE 8.4

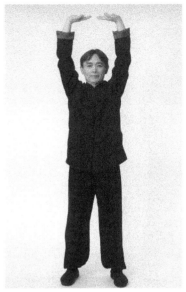

FIGURE 8.5

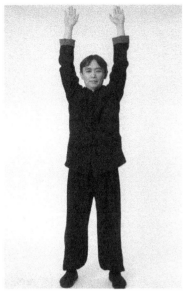

FIGURE 8.6

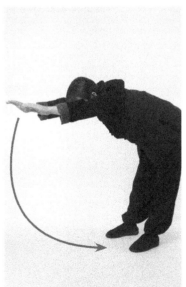

FIGURE 8.7

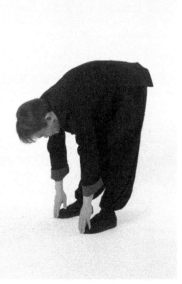

FIGURE 8.8

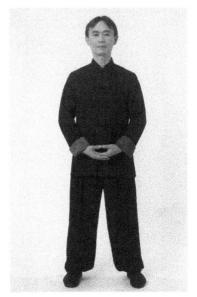

FIGURE 8.2